DIABULIMIA:

Towards Understanding, Recognition, And Healing

Aarti Sharma

For
my parents (Rajiv and Miriam), brother (Vikram), and aunt (Shobha)
whose unconditional love, support, and insight
have always granted me a an unshakeable faith in the future.

"For I know the plans I have for you," declares the Lord,
"plans to prosper you and not to harm you, plans to give you hope and a
future."
- Jeremiah 29:11

CONTENTS

PRELIMINARY NOTE

Diabulimia: Towards Understanding, Recognition, and Healing is generally intended for all audiences – patients, families, clinicians, and the curious academician or layman – in order to dissect, inform, narrate, and recommend. The book combines evidence-based and clinical facts, incorporating information from the medical/scientific literature whenever available. Other description is sourced from 1.) clinical anecdote via healthcare professionals in the field, 2.) patient interviews, and/or 3.) personal experience. Indeed, we must underscore that due to the paucity of research on the topic, much of the information contained herein is derived from the latter three aforementioned sources. Although the body of research is accruing slowly, we cannot yet endorse this as a collection of validated work but rather observations and attestations of clinical/social experience.

In order to serve the wide range of readers, there are sections unsuitable for specific populations. The incipient purpose was not for a single individual to comprehensively tackle the material; rather, we encourage the reader to select the segments which are most germane to their area of expertise or interest. Some chapters are highly technically/scientifically oriented, and others intended for a layman audience. Of course, perusing other chapters outside your realm of interest is useful for overall education, but do not let them become an impediment to those most particularly pertinent.

If you are a patient currently (or potentially, previously) suffering from the condition, we would strongly encourage you to proceed with caution. There are sections which might be triggering depending on your stage of physical recovery and psychological stability. Explicit methods of execution, narratives, statistics, numbers – any of which are dangerous – are examined here, so please do not let the material jeopardize your healing or continued recovery in any way. It is better that you close this volume immediately if you harbor even an inkling of reservation.

You will perhaps find it useful to tailor your reading based on the following chapter descriptions and recommendations:

Chapter 1: <u>Name</u> – General history of and introduction to diabulimia.

1

Chapter 2: <u>Behavioral Etiology</u> – Description of factors contributing to development of the illness; recommended for all audiences.

Chapter 3: <u>Pathophysiology</u> – Technical discussion of underlying molecular mechanisms of diabulimia; recommended only for those with medical/scientific background.

Chapter 4: <u>Characteristics</u> – Description of insulin patterns, epidemiology, observations made at the clinical appointment, and laboratory values. Intended more for the clinician, but also useful for the general public for recognition purposes.

Chapter 5: <u>Execution</u> – Examination of methodologies by which the patient with diabulimia might conceal their illness. Important for *both* the general public and clinician. Current patients should bypass this chapter.

Chapter 6: <u>Screening and Prevention</u> – Includes techniques by which diabulimia is elucidated; geared more towards the clinician.

Chapter 7: <u>Sequelae</u> – Potential physical and psychological consequences of diabulimia are described. Clinicians are most likely aware of these outside the context of diabulimia; intended more for the general public.

Chapter 8: <u>Treatment</u> – Comprehensive overview of diabulimia treatment approaches; recommended for all audiences.

Chapter 9: <u>Relapse</u> – Defines and expounds upon factors contributing to diabulimia reappearance; recommended for all audiences.

Chapter 10: <u>Living with Diabulimia</u> – Fictional narratives derived from field interviews. A literary shortcut towards internalizing some common symptoms and red flags of diabulimia; recommended for the general public and optional for the clinician.

Unfortunately, this volume only covers a tip of the diabulimia iceberg. There are many more details, frames of reference, and insights to be addressed, and we apologize for whatever deficits are present. But if *Diabulimia: Towards Understanding, Recognition, and Healing* enlightens even one patient, doctor, or family member, then our work has been accomplished.

INTRODUCTION

Diabetes – above all else – is a noun. It is said that Type I Diabetes is not a 'disease,' neither is it an 'illness,' nor a 'condition.' It is a lifestyle. But it is also a verb, an adjective, a predicate. It governs those nuances of life whose existences are deemed superfluous, irrelevant; it interdigitates through discomfort as well as calm. Diabetes is in no morphology poetic or romantically distressful; it can be humorous – but often at the prerequisite of satire.

Diabetes is a despot – and 'benevolent' here is irrelevant. His reign is earmarked by coup d'etats, by mutinies, by transient battles – where sometimes he is *le victoire,* and at other times his face is ground into the sand. He is never completely defeated – but fortunately that qualification does, and always will, apply to his opponent.

Testament to both its increasing prevalence, the public zeitgeist, and the contemporary standard of medical care, the diagnosis of Type I diabetes is not now considered as a figurative or literal death sentence. Patients – who half a century ago might have despaired for life and livelihood – now confront the news with an unprecedented margin of hope. This is due to a plethora of factors – the research sweeping the scientific world in all aspects of diabetes, the potential for a 'cure' (or concepts and materials closely matching its definition), the overwhelming volume of public support and education available through the internet, non-profit organizations, and personal contacts. There is a quietly pervading susurrus that Type I diabetes is on its last legs, that his sway of terror is on the verge of truckling to such a comprehensive opposition, that the definitive domino is soon set to topple in its sequential ferocity.

But there is a group that has been abandoned in the dust. Unknown amidst the majority, forgotten when left behind.

Those who are shackled by both the lack of knowledge about and dearth of treatment for their condition, those who see the signature on the lease for lethal complications penned by their own ambivalent hands. Those who understand in painful certainty what their bodies are undergoing, but who are nigh incapable of helping themselves. Those who see themselves spiraling into handicap, who reach out reticently for help – but withdraw after witnessing the stigmatic reception and uncomprehending ears.

These are the patients with diabulimia.

Part I

TOWARDS UNDERSTANDING

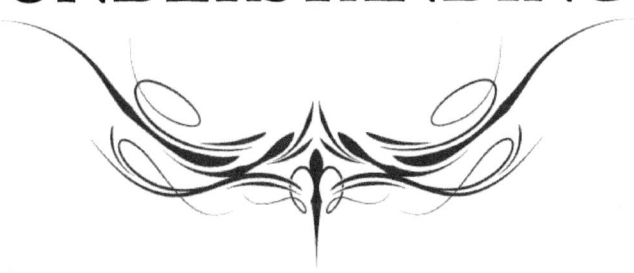

CHAPTER 1

NAME

But wait — there are actually some weak analogies, some metaphors of rhetoric which might suffice... Cancer, they sometimes say, "eats you from the inside out, both literally and figuratively — gnawing away at your organs, your emotions, your equanimity..." Diabulimia is the same. It's the same — except you're the one eating yourself from the inside out, wringing your brain and your body with your own recalcitrant hands. It's like being a drug addict, too, where you tell yourself one morning that it's okay, you can defeat this, you can defeat this, you can defeat this. *But the next day it's the old tired story, and you find yourself repeating the same hollow words in the twilight, where they resonate mockingly through your conflicted determination. You sorrow under the sun for preserving your body, and rejoice in the darkness while tearing it apart...recover for one day, and drown for a hundred. If you learn how to walk again, its breath will still be enticingly warm and toxic, whispering, beckoning — do we know any better but to succumb, are we encouraged differently, are we histrionically grabbed by the collar and yanked back into sensibility? Into life?*

No. We invented this illness. We exploit it. We perpetuate it. We kick it into the dust, we crawl back for forgiveness. We prevent our own healing. We search desperately for redemption. We plead to be unshackled.

But we ourselves have swallowed the keys.

W hat is diabulimia?

For the purposes of simple introduction – "diabulimia" by name is a fusion of the two words "diabetes" and "bulimia." Originally coined to convey the purging characteristic of bulimia nervosa, "diabulimia" stripped to its starkest definition is the 'use' of diabetes (most frequently Type I) to eliminate unwanted calories or weight. Unfortunately, the opportune phonetic continuity of the two words is rather a limiting factor in characterizing this condition. People hear the term "bulimia" and automatically visualize pathological vomiting or laxative use for weight control. Hence, they assume that "diabulimia" is simply the state of a patient with diabetes who concurrently suffers from bulimia nervosa. This is far from what the term is intended to relay.

As a short medical synopsis, Type I juvenile diabetes mellitus is characterized by autoimmune destruction or impairment of pancreatic beta-cells, which normally secrete the hormone insulin in order to regulate blood glucose concentration. In an insulin-dependent diabetic patient, these cells are generally destroyed or severely impaired before the age of 20, hence the term "juvenile." Patients are thenceforth required to normalize their blood glucose concentrations with exogenous insulin so to avoid the hazard of future complications consequent to hyperglycemia, including retinopathy, neuropathy, nephropathy, and cardiovascular malady.

Juvenile diabetes is diagnosed with [one or more of] glycosylated hemoglobin, random blood sugar, fasting blood glucose tests, and serum antibody levels against insulin-producing cells. The period prior to diagnosis is characterized by significant weight loss due to the body's inability to metabolize sugar, leading to elevated glucose levels (termed hyperglycemia). During this interval, the body resorts to breaking down muscle and fat for sustenance, creating a chronic state of ketoacidosis in which the brain adapts by utilizing ketone bodies instead of glucose as its primary fuel source. Hyperglycemia also induces an osmotic diuresis, forcing the body to excrete copious volumes of fluid. In addition, glucose (and its storage form glycogen) store four times their weight of water. As a consequence of both this diuretic effect and incapability to shelve glucose, the patient becomes dangerously dehydrated. The drastic weight loss prior to diagnosis is a combination of these two factors – significant expulsion of interstitial water, as well a literal cannibalization of tissue.

In essence, what the **P**atient **W**ith **D**iabulimia (henceforth abbreviated as "**PWDb**") seeks to recreate is this period prior to diagnosis for the primary purpose of controlling their weight. In psychological terms, the "inappropriate compensatory behavior" (mechanisms by which an individual with bulimia or anorexia nervosa attempts to rectify a recent binge episode) is the manipulation of insulin. This action is actually quite calculated, given the body's profound sensitivity to metabolic perturbations. If a diabetic patient eats a candy with a specific number of carbohydrates, and subsequently fails to provide themselves an appropriate amount of insulin, their blood sugar will rise. Above a blood sugar level of 180-200 mg/dl, the kidney's tubular capacity to reabsorb glucose becomes overwhelmed, resulting in glucose spillover into the urine. Below these levels all glucose in non-pathological states is completely reabsorbed back from the renal filtrate into the body. Classic symptoms of frequent urination and polydipsia consequently manifest in only a few hours. The mission then is essentially accomplished in the short-term: if the PWDb does not want that snack – unanticipated or otherwise – to translate into an extra inch of fat, they forego their insulin shot and (in gross essence) 'pee out the candy.'

Secondary to the deficiency of insulin, the body begins to produce ketone bodies from fatty acid oxidation within a few hours – which commences at non-pathological levels but under conditions of chronic insulin absence escalates to dangerous blood concentrations. Ketones are also renally eliminated, providing another micromolecular avenue of purging. *Essentially*, by transitivity: fats = ketones = ketonuria = 'urination of fat.'

Since the early 1970's, scientific publications and clinical studies have employed the phrase "eating disorder with insulin omission" in reference to the condition now known as diabulimia, but this usage has only perpetuated the medical and public perception that such an action is only an insignificant sequela of juvenile diabetes. Until recently, the lack of a concrete pathologic term has been a detriment to the condition as a whole – "insulin omission," while distinctive, is inept at providing recognition of the holistic illness especially as it relates to disturbed eating patterns. Unfortunately, efforts to rectify this situation are lackluster even today. For example, the Diagnostic and Statistical Manual of Mental Disorders IV, the standard reference for mental health professions, makes token allusion to insulin omission as medication manipulation for the purpose of weight loss as a behavioral disturbance associated with eating disorders: "[omission or reduction of] insulin doses in order to reduce the metabolism of food consumed during eating binges."[1] Unfortunately, this is far from adequate. It is no longer an exceptional practice, and must be understood and approached as such.[1(footnote)]

In order to address the particularities of insulin omission *for the purpose of weight control* as an eating disorder specific to patients with Type I diabetes, two terms have been propagated: "ED-DMT1 (Eating Disorders – Diabetes Mellitus Type I)," and, of course, "diabulimia." Even though the terminology of this particular illness has become somewhat of an alphabet

---

[1] As a matter of interest, another eating disorder analogous to diabulimia in that it also involves omission (and overconsumption) of medication for the purpose of weight control is the as-yet unnamed "thyroid bulimia." Endogenous and exogenous hyperthyroidisms inherently create a hypermetabolic state such that calories are utilized more rapidly and micromolecular energy substances have an elevated turnover rate. In fact, one of the presenting symptoms of the illness is conspicuous weight loss and heat intolerance, reflecting its thermogenic characteristics. As such, some patients abuse drugs prescribed for either acquired (i.e. thyroidectomy) or endogenous (autoimmune) hypothyroidism. They ingest the medication (levothyroxine, also known as Synthroid) in excess of their prescribed dosages so to enhance their metabolic furnace. By the same token, patients with endogenous hyperthyroidism (i.e. Graves disease) are usually treated with a drug termed methimazole (also known as Tapazole), which inhibits the synthesis of thyroid hormone. These patients fail to take adequate doses, leading again to a hyperthyroid state. This practice is not without its toxicities, however. Chronic hyperthyroidism has many deleterious effects, not the least of which are osteoporosis and cardiac arrhythmias. Patients can plausibly adapt to most of the initial symptoms, such as tachycardia, sweating, anxiety, and diarrhea, but generally become worried when their hair begins to fall out. This condition has its own distinctive characteristics, although the psychological similarities to diabulimia are uncanny. It requires another volume in itself.

soup, a discussion of the advantages and disadvantages of both as pertaining to both the clinical and laymen realms is warranted.

There are three distinct populations of patients relevant to this discussion, and they are often confused and/or conflated given the specificity of both eating disorder as well as insulin nomenclature/diagnostic criteria. These are 1.) diabetic patients without eating disorders, aka the 'control' or 'baseline' group referred to in clinical studies, 2.) diabetic patients with eating disorders without *intentional* insulin-omitting behaviors, and 3.) diabetic patients with eating disorders with *intentional* insulin-omitting behaviors. These can be further subdivided based on the types of compensatory behaviors and other parametrical details, but this is foregone for clarity.

Early in 2008, an international convention met in Minneapolis, Minnesota to confer an official inclusive nomenclature on the dual-diagnosis of Type I diabetes and an (or multiple) eating disorder/s: ED-DMT1 (Eating Disorder – Diabetes Mellitus Type 1).[2] Although this represents another step towards awareness, the taxonomy does little to parse "insulin omission" from the myriad contemporary disorders that eclipse it. The comorbidity of diabetes and eating disorders is detailed in a later chapter, but suffice it to say that this term lies on one extreme of the spectrum addressing insulin omission as a pathological tool for weight control. While it finally brings to the clinical eyepiece a prominent classification for illnesses which have thus far only been considered as 'correlations' or 'relationships,' ED-DMT1 is yet more of a category than it is a definitive term for the exact pathology we address here. If, for example, a patient is referred to a mental health professional as having "ED-DMT1," the name does little more to enlighten the clinician as to the precise pathology than describing the patient as a "Type I diabetic with an eating disorder." Do they manifest restrictive behavior typical of anorexia nervosa, or binge-purging behavior characteristic of bulimia nervosa? More importantly, are they practicing insulin restriction as a result of their psychopathology regarding food and/or weight? What other compensatory behaviors have they adopted along the chronology of diabetes and disordered eating? Despite its noble mission to encompass, the ambiguity of the term is innately confounding. It labors under the perilous misconception that Groups 2 and 3 should be combined under the same

11

canopy, when they are in fact discrete. An eating-disordered Type I diabetic practicing insulin omission solely or in combination with other compensatory behaviors (Group 3) cannot be recognized or treated in the same fashion as an eating-disordered Type I diabetic who does not use insulin as a purging tool.

The second term, "diabulimia," has only recently emerged into the public light, and its birth was not long prior. It was a catchy and opportune word coined during roughly the same period in which the Internet and its blogosphere gained strong footholds in regards to information dissemination – primarily in the mid-to-early 2000's. The earliest use of the word was not medical in origin but rather among family members or peers with the condition, most likely an informal labeling for that coterie who found "insulin omission" or "manipulation" too cumbersome, too esoteric for feasible communication. Even now, the medical literature understandably shies from utilizing the word due to its layperson 'slang' connotations (not to mention some semantic inaccuracies).

Compared to "ED-DMT1" as a codification addressing *insulin omission* for the purpose of weight control, however, "diabulimia" appears to be more apt for the endeavor. The term 'diabulimia' is far less equivocal than its peer as relating to the matter of insulin manipulation and hence more useful clinically. It delineates a patient with diabetes suffering from both **a.) an eating disorder**, and **b.)** even though the name itself might not indicate such, the public definition of the term has evolved an embedded cognizance of the presence of **insulin manipulation.** Furthermore, it successfully separates Group 3 from Group 2, with the stipulation that it does not immediately differentiate between restrictive and bingeing behaviors. If not for anything other than recognition purposes, these characteristics are exactly what the medical world needs in order to address "insulin omission for the purpose of weight control." "Diabulimia" grants patients a discrete nomenclature to identify with, although duly subject to misinterpretation. Putting a label on a pathology is a powerful preliminary step towards support maneuvers and treatment approaches.

This is most definitely not to say that "diabulimia" is a perfect word for such circumstances, but perhaps 'lesser of two evils is a more appropriate justification. As per this definition, it is not an isolated condition (other methods of purging might be present under an eating disorder umbrella). The term entails confusion due to the use of "bulimia," which might be taken to mean 'bulimia nervosa' instead of the purging aspect of this condition. This is actually quite a significant impediment – some patients and health professionals deny the illness simply because they or their patient 'don't throw up.' While vomiting is certainly one of the most common purging methods of *bulimia nervosa,* it is not the only one and should not be confused with *insulin omission* as a purging method.) "Diabulimia" is criticized by experienced clinicians as sometimes being too specific, too simplistic, too reductionist – after all, why not use "dianorexia" (diabetes + anorexia)? These patients also can restrict calories like classic anorexia nervosa patients, instead of practicing the bingeing/overconsumption behaviors more typical of bulimia nervosa.

The unfavorable truth is that both terminologies do this patient demographic a significant disservice by both the implications they make and the particularities which they exclude, but ultimately we must extract ourselves from this semantic argument and elect a term.

As the web interface became available to a larger population, the word "diabulimia" quickly disseminated and acquired traction among those patients or people familiar with the features of the condition. It appeared sporadically in various diabetes-centered forums and as the focus of short articles written for public medical websites – but these were neither widely distributed nor comprehensive in content. They barely addressed the skeleton of diabulimia, and were generally written from the perspective of a news reporter – someone who 'knew a person' who was or had suffered from diabulimia, and who had done their cursory research into standard complications of high blood sugar. These snippets simply blanket-defined diabulimia as 'teenage girls not taking insulin in order to lose weight, who can run into real problems in the future because of high blood sugar' which is – both holistically and specifically – a gross oversimplification of the actual condition. Some were judgmental in tone, others were objectively concerned, but few to none were more than statements of myopic information. There was no call to action, no mobilization of forces, no conviction. It was as if diabulimia was analogous to the latest celebrity scandal in the supermarket tabloids – shocking and fascinating but something to pass conveniently in one ear and out the other. Parents and families who were actively engaged in diabetes communities heard about this frightening 'new' illness in young diabetic girls, but either scoffed at such an outrageous idea, or – out of fear that their child might adopt such behaviors – silenced the concept into oblivion. Diabulimia was a serpentine whisper, attacking the vulnerable and slithering away from those who might have impeded its dissemination. Such lack of adhesion was manifest in not only the realm of the layman, but of the physician as well.

The era of both the social networking website (Facebook, Myspace) and the blogosphere witnessed the true emergence of diabulimia into both the private as well as public consciousness. These vehicles were the startling catalyst of diabulimia awareness, and the movement even today is on its training wheels. The creation of online communities and support groups through these avenues, combined with the ability to propagate personal narrative to an international audience, was instrumental in generating the current level of public knowledge germane to the condition. (It is not clear whether this availability – while obviously tremendously helpful towards increasing consciousness – is also perpetuating the illness.) Unfortunately, the proportion of clinicians knowledgeable about the condition has not accrued analogously.

Treatment centers for eating disorders originally were mystified as to how to effectively treat diabulimia, most not even comprehending the condition's gravitas. Patients have testified that available therapy was largely ineffective – bordering on insulting – as clinicians were unable to digest the idea that people would purposefully manipulate insulin for such 'frivolous' purposes. However, the past few years have seen an increase in the admission of patients with diabetes to eating disorder rehabilitation centers such as the Center for Hope of the Sierras in Reno, the Renfrew Center in Florida, and the Park Nicollet Melrose Center in Minneapolis. Most facilities in general now have a rudimentary, if not working, knowledge of how to initiate treatment with patients suffering from an insulin-omitting pathology.

This atmosphere is where we find ourselves today.

CHAPTER 2

BEHAVIORAL ETIOLOGY

To say that my life changed after being diagnosed with Type I borders on trite. I will only mention that in an already morose adolescent phase of my life, my own perception of self-tragedy was exacerbated by the fact that I could no longer be a 'normal' girl. I was placed on the standard regimen of blood sugar monitoring, insulin shots, and parental regulations. Thus for the first few years, my parents managed all of 'diabetes,' a situation for which I developed an exquisite sense of resentment. Rebellious as I was, there was simply no way to circumvent the glucose testing and insulin shots, the specific times of eating and the particularly tasty victuals I was discouraged or restricted from eating.

I never really cared about my weight before seeing how skinny I had become prior to diagnosis. In a way, I always resented the hospital for causing me to gain back all of that mass — I thought if they hadn't pumped me so chock-full of saline then I might still be thin. I would look at myself in the mirror and think, "I looked better all those months ago before diabetes." I'd cock my head in momentary retrospect, but I never dwelt on it.

At some point, though, these two things conflated. Somehow, along the way, I realized something which I thought made me inordinately clever. If I didn't take my insulin, I could eat whatever, whenever, and wherever I wanted. It was as simple as that. I didn't know enough about physiology yet to understand the concept of ketones or acidosis or glycosylated hemoglobin or glucose oxidation. I didn't even know what bulimia was, really. All I knew was that as long as my body was deprived of insulin, the glucose couldn't enter my muscles, and would remain in my bloodstream and eventually exit through my urine. It was a magical working manifesto for me — almost better than not having diabetes at all...

Towards Understanding

In the interest of prevention, we ask first how to nip the offending growth at the bud, before it has the chance to infiltrate the entire organism. So we inquire: "What is the cause of diabulimia? What is its activator?" If we seek to delve deeper, we ask, "How is the pathogenesis of diabulimia different from that of an eating disorder without insulin omission?" Or "What is the primary motive for omitting insulin – to lose weight, or negate the effects of food consumption, or both?"

The public definition of "diabulimia," unfortunately, has not evolved in parallel with the clinical categorization of eating disorders. The common understanding of diabulimia involves insulin omission at the center, and other factors (e.g., disturbed eating) as radii. However, for many health professionals, "diabulimia" as insulin-omission-for-weight-control is viewed under the lens of one of two major eating disorders: anorexia or bulimia nervosas (and occasionally EDNOS, or Eating Disorder Not Otherwise Specified). Therefore, there is a certain circularity inherent to the term "diabulimia" depending on the angle from which it is viewed. A majority of our analyses will draw upon the former perspective – with diabulimia at the center and other pathologies branching outward. At certain times, however, we will employ the other clinical perspective for clarity and classification – with insulin omission as a purging tool in the greater anorexia/bulimia/EDNOS context. Central to this type of analysis lies the tenet that if a patient practices insulin omission (Group 3 – refer to Chapter 1: page 11, and Figure 1 that follows), then they are also likely to present with other purging behaviors and a spectrum of disordered eating. This is regrettably a major derivative of Group 2's powerful and dangerous ability to obscure Group 3.

However, describing diabulimia as a *theoretically* separate pathology is extremely important, due to major characteristic differences described later in this chapter. This theoretical stance most closely resembles the public understanding of the illness – namely, that insulin omission is at the core, and concomitant pathologies are subclassifications of this action.

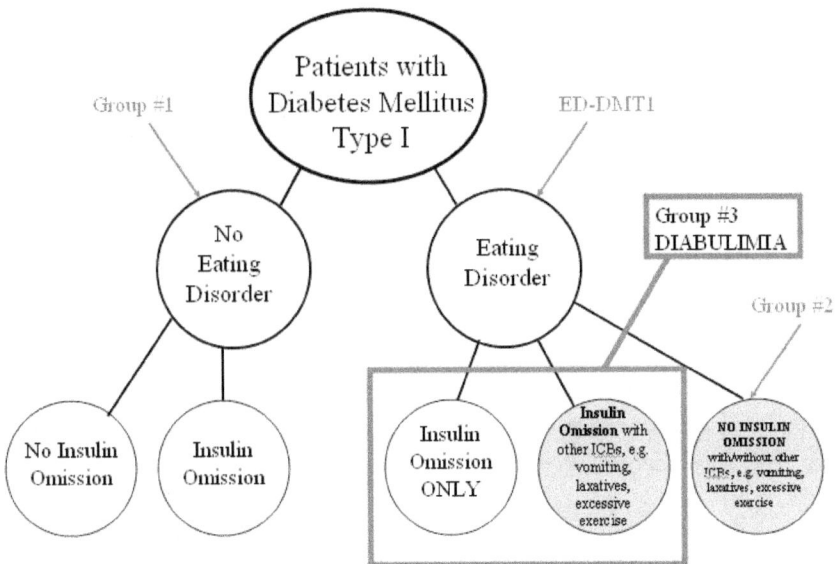

Figure 1: *This diagram illustrates further the subdivisions present under the diabetes and eating disorder canopy. (Sizes of circles are not proportional to respective prevalence.) Insulin omission also occurs without express existence of a cognitive eating disorder, as shown in the circles on the left side. Groups 1, 2, and 3 as they are described on page 11 are also indicated in this figure (arrows). The rightmost two capsules are shaded in grey to indicate the oft-blending of these distinct populations. Note that Group 3 includes both factions practicing insulin omission as a sole form of purging as well as those who use it in combination with other compensatory behaviors. Also note that ED-DMT1 encompasses all three capsules on the bottom right side of the figure. The word "diabulimia" in the vernacular signifies both "Insulin Omission ONLY," as well as "Insulin Omission with other ICB's." (Sometimes Group I patients- usually younger – can present to clinic with high HbA1c levels or to the ED with ketoacidosis after "not feeling like taking insulin for a few days" due simply to frustration with the stressful Type I diabetes lifestyle and other factors. This is **not diabulimia** as we have defined – it does not entail designs toward weight control. We can thus easily understand the confusion generated by the terminology surrounding this illness.*

The word 'cause' is inherently vague in regards to eating disorders, and not entirely useful for the purposes of this discussion. Purporting to pinpoint one precise cause is completely futile; in fact, consensus states that such an entity does not even exist. Let us therefore address 1.) 'susceptibilities' – those characteristics present in an individual's genetic/personality blueprint, 2.) 'triggers' – entities or a combination of entities that are immediate external activators of the abnormal behaviors, and 3.) 'motivation' – underlying dynamics intrinsic to the perpetuation or manifestation of the condition.

Both the 'susceptibility' and 'motivation' of diabulimia are highly complex, but they are, however, very similar to those of any other non-insulin-omitting eating disorder. In the apt words of one 22-year-old patient: *"Come to think of it, the eating disorder would have happened whether or not we had diabetes. It's a deep seed within us, you see, and diabetes simply gave us more awareness, more drive, and a convenient instrument with which to carry it out..."*

Research has demonstrated that genetic/epigenetic and physiological factors (e.g., neurotransmitter derangement) make certain individuals more likely to experience or engage in the prequels to eating disorder development. Certain psychological/personality traits, such as perfectionism, obsessive-compulsive, anxiety, mood, and borderline personality disorders, are also implicated. Family history, whether it entails an eating disorder in a parent or a predilection towards obesity, can also contribute. The combination of these variables renders some individuals more vulnerable to aberrations concerning food and body image.

Likewise, the mental provenance of eating disorders can often be traced to preoccupations with/intense focus on weight, shape, and personal appearance (body dysmorphia), and anxiety about/fixation on food, calories, and diet. They might allocate disproportionate amounts of self-worth on body image and/or consumption control, and manifest intense fear about gaining weight. These "motives" can claim contributions from environmental pressures to be thin/perfect/attractive, or they might arise from family dysfunction, adverse rebellious attitudes, sexual abuse, neurotransmitter derangement, and sequelae of other chronic illnesses, such as depression or injury.

The patient's 'trigger' might range from seeing an image of food, eating something they themselves have prohibited, hearing a remark about their weight, being in stressful situations, losing control over circumstances, feeling depressed, angry, lonely, nervous, insecure, even exhilarated or triumphant. The laundry list is regrettably infinite, and insulin omission might serve as a potent coping mechanism for any of these circumstances. We can in no way do complete justice to the torturous complexity of eating disorder etiology – susceptibilities, motivations, and triggers all integrate within different patients in different manners in order to generate these symptomatic abnormalities. Volumes can and have been written on such subjects alone.

Unfortunately, the presence of Type I diabetes only appends a much deeper level of psychopathology – lending patients a higher probability of developing disordered eating than their normal peers. This is one reason why it is so crucial that "diabulimia" be resolved from other "inappropriate compensatory behaviors" and general symptoms of eating disorders. It involves a completely discrete demographic with markedly different psychological baselines, an exclusive method of weight control, and even distinct impetuses (which will be enumerated below).

Type I Diabetes and Comorbidity of Eating Disorders

Let us first consider Group 2 (diabetic patients with eating disorders without insulin omission). Even the most cursory scan of the literature will reveal a prominently documented comorbidity of diabetes and eating disorders - *without considering diabulimia/insulin restriction specifically.* Many studies have shown that this coincidence is greater than what might be feasibly expected by chance, with as much as a 35% overlap.[1, 26] Incidentally, this 'dual-diagnosis' of diabetes and eating disorders – ED-DMT1, if you will – reveals considerably worse glycemic management upon long-term monitoring.[2-4] Although the two are not necessarily contingent, the frequency of their correlation is alarming and demands attention. Eating disorders induce both chronic hyperglycemia and hypoglycemia by virtue of diurnal irregularities and unpredictable food intake patterns. And the considerable dangers that arise when diabetics take inattentive care of blood glucose, whether intentionally or unintentionally, are common knowledge. In fact, in a study performed by Steel et al. (1987), only four out of fifteen patients with eating disorders did not have microvascular complications secondary to poor metabolic control, in stark comparison with the prevalence of complications incurred by Type I diabetic patients without eating disorders.[7] Other sequelae include nephropathy, neuropathy, and even mortality.

In multiple cases of bulimia nervosa, binge-eating disorder, and anorexia nervosa, the long-term glucose values (measured by glycosylated hemoglobin, or HbA1c values) of Type I diabetic patients were dramatically elevated.[5,6] An eating disordered patient can quite feasibly have chronically high blood sugars even if they administer what they sincerely believe are correct insulin doses. Disordered eating innately perpetuates hyperglycemia through *both* accidental hiatus/lack of appropriate dosing for irregular meals and/or the deliberate neglect of such therapy.[8-10] Insulin omission is in fact one of the most common purging methods for ED-DMT1 patients, and *this* action in *this particular population* that specifically constitutes 'diabulimia.'

What, then, makes these patients so vulnerable – perhaps more so than the general population – to the development of eating disorders?

The diagnosis of Type I diabetes itself, is, first and foremost, a powerful source of psychological trauma. While in many patients this disturbance never attains clinical significance as disorders of anxiety/post-traumatic/acute stress/adjustment, it is nevertheless a potent underlying cause of many cognitive aberrations. It represents a profound perturbation of the patient's perceptions regarding the natural order of their environment, leaving them vulnerable and mentally insecure. In Type I diabetes especially, this trauma might not manifest immediately due to the urgent and overwhelming volume of material that the patient must not only internalize but effectively begin to execute within the space of a few days and weeks. Adaptation to life with Type I is not trivial; the illness almost literally permeates and alters every nuance of a patient's existence. This concurrent level of stress might obscure any potential injury induced by the diagnosis itself, which manifests as delayed repercussions. Indeed, one of the most common and compelling sources of eating disorders is trauma of this psychological grade. As mentioned, however, many patients can adjust to a new baseline with minor evidence of perturbance or displacement.

The Diagnostic and Statistical Manual of Mental Disorders, 4th edition (DSM-IV) system of analysis is multi-axial, incorporating many facets of an individual's existence so as to address the psychiatric pathology in an overarching context. It consists of 5 axes enumerating the principal disorder (axis I), concomitant personality disorders (II), medical problems (III), psychosocial stressors (IV), and global functioning (V). Given that the principal disorder (axis I) is an eating pathology, the two axes most important (within our particular context) are medical problems (axis III) and psychosocial stressors (axis IV). The chronic presence of Type I diabetes qualifies as an axis III inclusion, and the acute diagnosis of or sequelae associated with diabetes management are included in axis IV. Given this predisposing baseline, the presence of diabetes almost by default lays an insidious framework for the development of psychiatric pathologies. (The recently released DSM-V has abandoned the multiaxial system, but many major institutions still utilize the definitions in this transitional period.)

Furthermore, many patients are diagnosed at precisely the 'opportune' age to develop diabulimia, namely those formative peri-adolescent years. This combination of entering/exiting puberty and being diagnosed with diabetes for many patients influences the factors contributing towards disordered eating.[25] Puberty already compromises the patient's sense of control given the myriad transformations and transitions occurring during this formative period (e.g. hormonal, emotional, and bodily changes, tapering of parental influence, greater social emphasis on peer opinion). Along comes diabetes to wrench away any vestige of apparent autonomy. The fact that the diagnosis is often idiopathic only intensifies any accompanying frustration.

Next, numerous external changes manifest in a diabetic body immediately post-diagnosis, which might "trigger" an already susceptible mind or induce malaise in those as-yet untainted. For reasons to be discussed later, there is an abrupt and (overtly) irreversible weight gain following reinstitution of insulin therapy – primarily fluid retention manifesting as peripheral edema. Not uncommonly, newly-diagnosed patients gain 5-10 lbs in the hospital after saline rehydration, followed by another 5-10 lbs during successive days. Considering the striking weight loss that occurs pre-diagnosis, a reverse *gain* of 10-20 lbs (albeit largely non-pathological) above their original baseline is alarming even to a mind not attuned to body mass. This phenomenon leaves the adolescent diabetic dangerously vulnerable to disruptive eating patterns designed to revert to their previous body mass indices.[11,12]

During the pre-diagnosis state, the body also cannibalizes an appreciable amount of lean muscle tissue – those cells which contribute a major percentage of the basal and resting metabolic rates. Upon reinstitution of therapy, this foregone muscle mass translates into a curtailed caloric requirement, which leaves the patient more prone to weight gain. In combination with the post-normoglycemic fluid retention, this compounds the patient's already potentially distorted view concerning weight and eating.[13]

Patients also typically gain weight with intensive insulin therapy (water retention notwithstanding) which contributes to the relatively higher weights of many Type I diabetics. Data suggests a 33% increase in risk that diabetics become overweight or obese after intensive insulin care as opposed to 9.3% increase who undergo conventional treatment.[14] Efforts toward tighter blood sugar management also statistically increase the occurrence of hypoglycemic excursions. During these episodes, patients must consume extra sugar to rectify the low blood sugar levels. Unfortunately, given the inadequate glucose supplying the brain, patients feel confused and inordinately hungry, leading to caloric consumption oftentimes greater than their overall somatic requirement for blood sugar normalization. This, needless to say, can result in higher body mass over a period of time. And yet further – not that any additional evidence is qualitatively required to prove this point – one of the key features of undiagnosed Type I diabetes is polyphagia (excessive somatic-induced eating), such that the amount ingested can be twice to thrice the caloric requirement of a normal adult. Post-diagnosis, some patients find difficultly in drastically reducing their intake while conforming to their true metabolic rate. Weight gain ensues consequent to the perpetuated excess.

Anorexia nervosa and bulimia nervosa in the non-diabetic population are frequently rendered susceptible, motivated, and triggered by atypical relationships toward food and eating, and the combination of these two factors. They develop in some cases by fixation on caloric and macronutritional content, preparation of foods, preoccupation with the timing, speed, and manner of eating, or any permutation thereof. While this is usually pathological in the general population, these are cognitions faced – sometimes necessarily – by the diabetic patient on a daily basis. Proper metabolic control requires knowing the carbohydrate content of every bite ingested, the timing of insulin dosing in relation to the lapse since the last repast, and generally many other variables concerning the two overarching parameters of food and eating. It is a marginally iatrogenic problem, sometimes further exacerbated in younger patients whose parents/guardians constantly monitor diet, hone insulin dosing and carbohydrate counting down to a science, and limit their diabetic child's intake of certain pleasurable foods. Diabetic patients are also at an earlier age (or earlier in life than would otherwise warrant) inculcated with the concepts of 'healthy weight and exercise' as these generally improve glucose management. It is not surprising then, given this incessantly and requisitely elevated awareness, that Type I diabetic patients are more prone to disordered eating behaviors.

Some theories attribute the greater momentum behind both insulin and non-insulin-omitting eating disorders to the adolescent diabetic's conscious deprivation of food despite hunger signals, due to the necessity of adhering to limited eating times/foods for maximal blood glucose control. This is a spearhead into binge eating and other dietary anomaly, catalyzed by a breach in these dietary constraints (what is termed the 'abstinence-violation' effect).[19, 27] Poor glycemic management and any type of disordered eating are virtually inseparable – once a normal pattern of caloric ingestion is relinquished, the routine of insulin use is likewise abandoned. This is especially evident in disorders entailing excessive consumption of food, namely bulimia nervosa and binge-eating disorder. Whether an episode of overeating is sparked by hypoglycemia or an environmental insult, the ensuing feelings of inadequacy and loss of control (among others) in these diabetics often stimulate the simplest ICB available: "metabolic purging" through skipping insulin doses. However, we mention again that the presence of disordered eating combined with chronic hyperglycemia does not automatically indicate diabulimia – patients dosing themselves with what they genuinely believe to be proper amounts of insulin might still grossly miscalculate dosages due to these dietary aberrations. For example, well-intentioned diabetic patients with binge-eating disorder (which by definition does not entail a purging mechanism, thereby technically eliminating intentional insulin omission/diabulimia) still have suboptimal metabolic control due to the difficulty involved in calculating insulin doses post-binge. In a study performed by Takii et al., (1999) comparing Type I patients with either bulimia nervosa or binge-eating disorder, patients with bulimia had statistically higher HbA1c levels and a greater rate of microvascular complications of hyperglycemia. This suggests that the above metabolic sequelae can be attributed more to concomitant insulin manipulation in the bulimia subgroup (occurring in 73%) rather than the type or quantity of food ingested during the binge episodes.[16]

On the opposite end of the spectrum, Type I diabetes and its grueling demand for blood sugar maintenance can induce undereating (sometimes to pathological extents). This pattern is more cognitively controlled (compared with overeating/bingeing), as patients might attempt to reduce the strenuousness of their diabetes regimen simply by willfully restricting consumption. By virtue of decreasing intake, the patient is liberated from the time and effort spent on insulin dosing and blood sugar monitoring, .while still maintaining proper glycemic levels. Unfortunately, the concomitant cognitive notations concerning control, infallibility, and invincibility resulting from 'freedom,' weight loss, and good diabetes management elevate the decreased consumption to pathological levels. They simultaneously warp the patient's psychology such that what was once a marginally harmless intention to control blood sugar now evolves into an attempt to control weight, shape, and circumstances. The patient can also present at the onset with anorexia nervosa *without* insulin omission, but for the reasons described throughout this chapter, can very plausibly adopt such behaviors.

DIABULIMIA:
Type I Diabetes + Eating Disorder + Insulin Omission

Patients have narrated on multiple occasions – both at the onset of diabulimia, and in ongoing recoveries/recurrences – that even minor insulin omission powerfully instigates full-blown pathology. The episode begins with innocuous mentations such as "I just won't take my shots for a week so I can drop a few pounds – after that I'll go right back," or "I really don't want that huge dinner to stick to my waist, I'll run high tonight and then correct tomorrow afternoon," which almost inevitably escalate to chronic hyperglycemia if allowed protraction. More often than not, this is exactly what happens – aberrant thoughts regarding weight/food/shape become cognitively entrenched, and the small amounts of insulin restriction provide strong positive reinforcement in the literal morphology of rapid weight loss. (Water excretion constitutes a majority, but this is hardly recognizable to a patient consumed by distorted thinking regarding body mass/eating/shape). Despite its bland tone, omitting "a few units" is actually enormously perilous. The development of other inappropriate compensatory behaviors, such as vomiting and diuretic use, might also ensue if not already present,[4] and this array promotes advancement of other, well-recognized psychiatric pathologies, including distress (both diabetes-specific and general emotional), depression, and neurosis.[17,18] Insulin omission is reported to occur in as many as 50% of Type I patients with a clinical or subthreshold eating disorder. A 2002 Scandinavian meta-analysis reported a notably elevated odds ratio (of 12) of eating disorders and the subsequent development of insulin misuse.[24]

Essentially, the PWDb places unreasonable worth on their attitude towards weight/food/shape such that they consciously elect to ignore the concurrent and inevitable destruction to their bodies. Some describe this as a sensation of invincibility, of defeating inevitable weight gain, of embracing the perception that nothing crippling will ever come to fruition. Outside parties (family, friends, insurance companies) find difficulty in comprehending this overall etiology. People do not and cannot appreciate the fact that a patient with diabulimia does not simply wake up one morning and decide to 'give themselves insulin.' The psychopathology is too insidious and exquisitely ingrained for such simplistic and streamlined reparation; unfortunately such complexity is not evident to anyone who has not experienced the condition firsthand or had extensive contact with patients under its chokehold.

Diabulimia can itself evolve to become the trigger and motivation of the eating disorder, creating a vicious cycle of negative reinforcement.

Towards Understanding

The condition becomes so indelible that it creates similar factors as those inducing the eating disorder in the first place. The apparent inability to conquer the illness sources distress, anxiety, and depression, which leads to either 1.) exacerbation of insulin restriction/disturbed eating, or 2.) relapse during an interval of potential remission. While before it might have been the symptomatic manifestation of other adverse neuropsychiatric processes, diabulimia soon becomes a component of these processes themselves in a cruel feedback system. The patient becomes entangled in a cycle of self-fulfilling prophecy, where their own discouraging convictions concerning recovery, guilt, and self-esteem abet further entrenchment of the same beliefs. Stated simply – diabulimia eventually causes diabulimia, and the 'controller' becomes the 'controlled.'

Fear of hypoglycemia also presents a compelling underlying drive as well as a prospective catalyst. One of insulin's physiological roles (generally in the non-pathological absence of available calories) is to promote hunger signals independent of the immediate necessity for calories. When a diabetic patient becomes hypoglycemic, they experience a strong impetus for *caloric* – not just glucose – consumption. Unfortunately, due to hypoglycemic confusion and mental disorientation, they can ingest a volume of food above and beyond what is required for blood glucose normalization. This provides potential 'binge' ingression, which understandably incites mental repercussions during periods of normality – fear of weight gain, losing control, and such. The diabetic might thereafter experience anxiety with insulin administration due to apprehension concerning psychosomatic overeating, leading to underdosing or complete neglect thereof. Once such a pattern is initiated, it is difficult to correct and may continue unremittingly.

The provenance of both diabulimia and non-insulin-omitting eating disorders can also be a rebellion against authority in regards to insulin treatment. Preteen and adolescent diabetics commonly demonstrate strong recalcitrance and resentment towards the agent (parent/guardian) enforcing insulin shots, blood sugar testing, and food intake discipline – details with which people of this age do not want to be hounded. ("Teen rebellion," is the name adopted by and granted special significance within juvenile diabetic communities, given the issues that these unique adolescents must manage.) Consequently, they choose to 'act out' by abandoning or refusing compliance with their diabetes treatment. Along this already detrimental path, patients learn serendipitously that they are able to eat as much as they want and not gain weight, or even lose weight. For a person formerly restricted to eating delineated quantities and types of foods at specific times, the newfound realization of this freedom along with the windfalls of weight loss and uncontrolled intake virtually lay the proverbial yellow brick road to diabulimia.[2]

---

[2]   Proliferation of the internet and blogosphere in the past decade has played a role of controversial importance in providing both the "motivation" and "triggers" for diabulimia. The fecundity of the web has facilitated both access to and availability of certain images, which are adversely compelling both at face value and also when analyzed and assigned a worth. The idea that "the media abets eating disorders" is an unfortunate misconception (most people are exposed to the same propaganda yet do not develop these conditions). Nevertheless, the media does exploit potent psychological weaponry in eating disorder promotion. Representations of food in gory detail, painfully thin but aesthetized females, the glut of dietary advice pertaining to bodily figure – none inspire positive impressions. This ubiquitous information and imagery is especially powerful given that they embody articles and feelings from which diabetic patients are instructed to abstain or limit.

It is also quite possible that the greater sophistication and speed of communication via development of discussion forums, chat rooms, and instant messaging has contributed towards disseminating the "idea" of diabulimia. Even though the illness has been sporadically documented since the early 1970's (and was obviously practiced prior to documentation), the recent increase in incidence/prevalence is most likely a reflection in part of the greater efficiency of interpersonal and cybernetic contact. Cases in point are the so-called "pro-ana" and "pro-mia" websites, which profess to be online forums for the support, discussion, and even social/familial rationalization of anorexia nervosa and bulimia nervosa, respectively. While diabulimia has not yet reached this level of public affirmation (and hopefully never will), the potential is not insignificant. This premise of technological dissemination creates a regrettable predicament for those seeking to increase diabulimia awareness. These mediums are beneficial for PWDbs as they facilitate creation of fostering groups with faceted perspectives other than those generated by more elementary communicative forms. But is it actually counterproductive and/or possibly iatrogenic – are we perpetuating the condition by increasing awareness without discriminating between the general public and the vulnerable populations? Is it even possible to parse these? This conundrum remains to be answered, especially in light of the endeavor to help clinicians determine whether their patients are engaging in this type of behavior. Tactful screening and questioning must be employed if diabulimia is suspected so as not to carelessly and inadvertently "advertise" this dangerous (and potentially lethal) technique of weight control.

Other diabetes-specific factors, including 1.) inability to afford insulin secondary to healthcare or employment disturbances, and 2.) distress and fears of the following: extraneous attention, hypoglycemia, and needles, might also contribute to insulin omission and should be distinguished from misuse only for the purpose of weight control. (Refer to Figure 1, Group #1.) This would therefore *not* fulfill our definition of "diabulimia." Patients might also feel that insulin use directly induces the depressive emotions concurrent with the diabetes lifestyle, and forego it in an attempt to mollify such feelings. Those skipping insulin for the sake of these factors had significantly better (although still sub-optimal) glycemic control than those neglecting their treatments for the purpose of weight control. Although insulin omission due to these diabetes-specific factors appears similar to omission for the purpose of rebellion in that neither of them is expressly intended for the purpose of weight control, omission to rebel against authority produces worse effects upon follow-up, and results in more consequential diabulimia as measured by the glycosylated hemoglobin level.[15]

We must note here that although there are a plethora of diabetes-specific contributions towards development of disordered eating, these are by no means the only etiologies. Other 'non-diabetic' circumstances, such as sexual abuse, family dysfunction, or environmental pressure, are as likely to contribute and cannot be excluded from the psychological assessment. Additionally, many of these factors are sufficient but not necessary (and vice versa) – lending credence to the principle that they are classically multifactorial in etiology. This explains why some people who are exposed to the same influences escape unscathed, while others progress to develop such pathologies. Unfortunately, as examined later, this deals a heavy blow to the concept of primary prevention.

The above discussion brings under examination the chronology of diabulimia progression, or the interval that generally passes after diagnosis for manifestation. There is no data available in the literature to suitably answer this question, so the evidence is anecdotal. The general observation between endocrinologists and psychiatrists is that diabulimia most frequently unfolds 2-3 years post-diagnosis.

However, due to the fact that insulin omission presents clinically with other compensatory behaviors, this might be too simplistic an inquiry. A more useful question addresses what proportion of patients who practice insulin omission also use other purging mechanisms, which of these compensatory behaviors are most prevalent, and when they manifested (i.e. before or after the Type I diagnosis). Data regarding this subject is again reported from clinicians, who generally testify that rarely do patients demonstrate insulin omission as their only mechanism of purging, and if it does present with other compensatory behaviors, emesis is usually the most prevalent. Concerning chronology, the patient might have suffered from a non-insulin-omitting eating disorder prior to diagnosis, which transformed into diabulimia after the onset of diabetes. That is to say, a member of Group 2 switches to Group 3 (referring to the distinctions made at the beginning of the chapter).

Separating diabulimia from a non-insulin-omitting eating disorder is no mean task if provided only clinical values and observations. Part of this difficulty is ascribed to perpetuated hyperglycemia through accidental hiatus/lack of appropriate dosing for irregular meals during disordered eating (without purposeful insulin omission). Compare the patient from Group 3 (eating disorder + insulin omission) with that from Group 2 (eating disorder without insulin omission). They will both typically present with elevated HbA1c levels in addition to similar somatic symptoms. At times, the only way to distinguish them is asking directly whether the patient is using insulin for a weight control endeavor. Some will question the clinical utility of separating the two, if the endocrinologist's ultimate goal is to normalize blood sugar levels and prevent end-organ damage. Unfortunately, the similarity in metabolic control between these two groups is largely a 'window period' in that Group 3: a.) lies on a far more precarious psychological baseline, b.) manifests symptoms which are guaranteed progression to acute crisis or chronic instability, c.) is more refractory to psychological and nutritional treatment. A similar problem arises when attempting to parse the non-eating-disordered patient who omits insulin through neglect (roughly, Group 1) for whatever reason – i.e., "I just let my insulin shots fall by the wayside for a while – didn't have time, didn't care, didn't remember." The same rationale used above for distinguishing Group 2 from Group 3 applies here – Group 1 is much more likely to be coaxed back into compliance and proper management due to their relatively unsullied cognitive framework.

Clinical detection is often confounded by virtue of this "overlap" effect, where the maintenance of non-insulin-manipulating ICBs post-diagnosis effectively equivocates the presence of diabulimia. Some PWDbs can 'sail by' through intentionally omitting only miniscule amounts of insulin, thus evading detection because the 'diabetic' transgression is successfully obscured by conventional purging methods. (These are more often the 'restrictive' pattern type of diabulimia patients, rather than the 'bingeing.' Caloric intake is curtailed to such an extent that requisite insulin is dramatically reduced – omission consequently has less of a deleterious effect than that for an individual with chronic/acute over-consumption patterns.[3]) Clinicians testify that patients engaging in insulin restriction in

---

[3]   There is a dietary pattern currently in practice by diabetic patients, bodybuilders, and individuals seeking to 1.) increase their lean mass, 2.) decrease adipose tissue, and 3.) improve their diabetes management. It is known as the high fat, low carbohydrate (HFLC) diet. We mention it here due to its confounding similarity to restrictive diabulimia patients, and the important principles that it highlights in relation to differentiating diabulimia from other, even nonpathological patterns. The philosophy of HFLC is such: lower levels of insulin, despite the presence of higher dietary fat, translates into decreased formation of adipose tissue. The intake calories are thereby shuttled towards more "aesthetic" areas/tissues (such as muscle) which is ideal for those seeking to lose weight as well as increase lean tissue. Decreased body fat and increased muscle mass has also been demonstrated to abet diabetes control by enhancing insulin sensitivity and decreasing total daily insulin requirements. Individuals adherent to HFLC partition their intake into high fat and restricted carbohydrates so as to enable themselves to dose less insulin *while still fully accounting for what is ingested.* It is a common and dangerous misconception that HFLC, by virtue of the fact that the diabetic intentionally "gives themselves less insulin" is synonymous to diabulimia. These individuals "restrict" their carbohydrates, *not* their insulin – viz., the insulin restriction is *secondary* to carbohydrate restriction, and patients still receive the appropriate doses. Diabulimia patients, on the other hand, DO NOT dose themselves properly for what is ingested, even though their carbohydrate intake might be similarly constrained (as is what frequently occurs in a restrictive PWDb). These patients consume so few carbohydrates that even omitting insulin will not result in salient hyperglycemia, which is why some of them can successfully escape detection due to relatively normal HbA1c levels. HFLC diets are useful to illustrate this important principle that diabulimia does NOT involve simplistically "low levels of insulin." It involves a *restriction, omission,* or *manipulation* of insulin totally *inappropriate for the corresponding amount of carbohydrates or calories ingested.*

fact typically present with a history of non-insulin-omitting eating disorders both before and after diagnosis. These then overlap with and continue in parallel with the diabulimia aspect of the overall medical situation. For example, a patient might have suffered from bulimia nervosa with vomiting/laxatives/excessive exercise/etc. before being diagnosed with diabetes, after which they began to omit insulin in addition to their original pattern of ICBs.

Furthermore, omission of insulin therapy is also not reserved for patients with full-fledged eating disorders.[20] Consumption of abnormal amounts of food, whether undereating or overeating, does not preclude calculated insulin manipulation, which is another factor in both misdiagnosis and absence of detection. Patients' eating habits might be completely acceptable but their purging actions through insulin neglect are no less alarming than conventionally disturbed eating patterns.[21, 22] Such subjects – often categorized as having 'subclinical' eating disorders (lacking an essential feature of a full-threshold condition) or 'eating disorder not otherwise specified' (EDNOS), also manifest poor glucose control. In one clinical study, the severity of the eating disorder – from inexistent, subclinical, to advanced – was found to correlate directly and even linearly with the magnitude of glycosylated hemoglobin values.[23] In fact, patients with EDNOS are at profound risk of developing a full-threshold eating disorder later in life, and should be perceived/approached as such (especially younger populations, in whom earlier recognition and treatment correlates with better prognosis for recovery). However, the unfortunate

---

A justifiable question arising from this distinction is why, then, to consider restrictive diabulimia as dangerous if it does not inherently generate aberrant glucose levels. The main concern lies in the psychopathology of the PWDb, and what such action could potentiate. (The peril of severe nutritional deficiency during restrictive behavior, even without insulin manipulation, goes without saying.) Here, the very *intention* to manipulate insulin is the differentiating factor – an already distorted idea which, despite the lack of quantifiable manifestation (i.e. HbA1c), is *not* innocuous. This intention is overarching and can progress to affect the PWDb's functioning and cognition. Physiological and psychological mechanisms during caloric restriction also unconsciously dictate the likely transition to bingeing behaviors, which is not an insignificant sequelae of anorexia nervosa. Omission during periods of restriction does not preclude omission during periods of bingeing or binge-restriction, and the PWDb might very well progress to intentional hyperglycemia if they continue to restrict their insulin following development of these behaviors.

consequence of this 'limbo' classification is that EDNOS patients receive suboptimal intervention due to their apparently benign presentation.

The existence of these multiple unconventional factors in Type I diabetes partially explains why there is a wide spectrum of presenting characteristics, to be discussed in later chapters. However, it is absolutely essential that clinicians and close familial/social contacts internalize the following axiom: the concept *and* execution of insulin omission for the purpose of weight control is *NOT* considered outlandish in the mind of the diabetic. It is a *frighteningly* logical outcome of very rational observations, computations, and conclusions. For the clinician especially: do not discount this in any relevant differential diagnosis.[4]

---

4   *"Diabulimia"* or "Eating Disorder...+ Insulin Omission"?

Given these classifications, it follows to question whether diabulimia should be considered a discrete pathology if it is just a mechanism of execution of anorexia nervosa or bulimia nervosa. After all, vomiting, laxative use, and excessive exercise are not generally considered as detached conditions but rather selectively exhibited elements/symptoms/patterns of a holistic illness. In other words, why should we not discuss diabulimia as part of its allocated place in the ICB aggregate instead of a transcendent condition?

This is a very valid point, and must be considered carefully especially in light of clinical proficiency. Must diabulimia – defined in its gross entirety as purposeful insulin manipulation motivated by weight control – in fact stand alone as a classified nomenclature? The perspective we adopt here is crucial: if we were to examine the PWDb from a mental health professional's frame of reference, our answer would be qualitatively negative. These physicians are trained to detect eating disorders and relatively more aware of insulin omission as a purging mechanism. However – and this is the primary problem of recognition facing us today – the mental health professional is not typically the first clinician coming into contact with the PWDb. The endocrinologist, members of the diabetic "team," and immediate familial/social contacts fulfill this role in the modern healthcare sequence for a Type I diabetic, and per contra, are not explicitly searching for the presence of eating disorders or intentional insulin restriction. Diabulimia must then be considered as an 'isolated' illness (not just a purging mechanism) when we survey the issue from the lens of a standard endocrinologist. Their context regarding this matter does not include the array of available eating disorder diagnoses but rather permutations of diabetes. As they are accustomed to treating aberrations of this pathology, understanding "diabulimia" to be discrete would dramatically increase awareness of *intentional insulin omission/weight control* as the problem to be addressed.

Behavioral Types of Diabulimia

We will also distinguish between two types of diabulimia, as they are both significantly different in both execution, pathophysiology, and clinical presentation. (Although they are almost never so starkly contrasted when demonstrated in reality, understanding the separate qualitative distinctions in the behavior underlying both is useful.)

1.) The first is a 'restrictive' type of diabulimia: the patient is limiting her intake of calories in combination with the omission of insulin (and perhaps by another ICB) in order to control weight.

2.) The second is a 'bingeing' type of diabulimia, where the patient consumes an excessive amount of calories and eliminates them by omitting insulin (and perhaps another ICB).

Both of these are defined here with the assumption of 'overall,' or 'most frequently,' as patients are not completely consistent in either their patterns of consumption or omission, existing rather along a spectrum.

Some might argue that other purging behaviors are frequently present in addition to insulin omission, and therefore "diabulimia" is too reductionist a concept for the physician setting. However, many times the most outstanding clues available to the diabetes clinician which indicate the presence of an *overall* eating disorder are those resulting directly from insulin omission, not the least of which are elevated glycosylated hemoglobin levels, lack of diabetes activity, and recurrent episodes of ketonuria/emergency ketoacidosis. For clinicians not specifically trained in the recognition of eating disorders, awareness of these diabulimia "red flags" might alert to the aggregate presence of bulimia or anorexia nervosa. Our rationale, then, for presenting insulin omission as theoretically independent throughout this book is for the salient differences in

- etiology/motivation
- clinical presentation
- execution
- longitudinal complications and mortality rates

between 1.) non-diabetic, 2.) diabetic eating-disordered patients *without* intended insulin omission, and 3.) diabetic eating disordered patients *with* intended insulin omission, i.e. diabulimia. It will intermittently seem that such terminology is circular, but this is only an artifact of the angle we have elected.

Towards Understanding

Some patients might alternate between the two forms, such that they become indistinguishable from each other. There might be cases in which there is a net loss of calories despite episodes of bingeing ('restrictive'), and vice versa, a net gain of calories despite episodes of caloric restriction ('binge/purging'). Anecdotally, the bingeing subtype of diabulimia is far more common.

The current categorization of non-insulin-omitting eating disorders is sometimes frustrating to understand, involving specific clinical criteria which can be confusing (for example, 'binge/purge' subtypes are involved in *both* bulimia and anorexia nervosas). We could also present these two diabulimia subtypes as anorexia nervosa or bulimia nervosa, respectively, with insulin omission as a purging tool. But that is not useful here. Our goal is to distinguish diabulimia from confounding/obscuring factors for didactic recognition purposes, and subsequently we present these 'subclassifications' of diabulimia as the outstanding pathologies themselves, rather than components of a pathology (i.e. ICBs for anorexia or bulimia nervosas). In reality, non-diabetic, non-insulin-omitting eating disorders themselves also present along a spectrum – patients do not absolutely conform to either bulimia or anorexia as per the clinical definitions, which were instituted more for research and codification purposes, with the majority of patients with eating disorders actually meeting diagnostic criteria for "Eating Disorder Not Otherwise Specified."

Factors underlying of the "restrictive" type of diabulimia pattern are attributed to a panoply of factors and attitudes relating to body image, food, and weight. Contrary to popular belief, anorexia nervosa in no way requires a mental unawareness of or aversion to food, and restrictive diabulimia by default is no different. Frequently these patients possess an exquisite and encyclopedic knowledge of nutrition and caloric content, and hold this cognizance as a proxy for actually consuming material food. In this way, they are able to convince themselves that they can control their weight, and persist in dieting and purging indefinitely. As such, PWDbs with restrictive patterns are usually described as ego-syntonic, namely that their behaviors, values, and impulses are generally compatible with their fundamental beliefs and characteristics. Discussing the variations of anorectic cognizance and behavior pertaining to food consumption and purging is beyond the scope of this book, but suffice it to say that throwing insulin omission into the bedlam only exacerbates distorted ideations.

Underlying incentives for "bingeing" diabulimia are not significantly different. As with bulimia nervosa, the purpose of purging (here, with insulin omission) is to mitigate the effects of caloric over-consumption. These episodes might be premeditated or completely unpredictable – in other words, the PWDb might intentionally and calculably overeat for a variety of reasons (which does not expressly qualify as a 'binge,') or on other hand the overconsumption might dictated by somatic factors (e.g. 'binge' episode). As such (in contrast to restrictive PWDbs), binge-purge patients are generally described as ego-dystonic. Although the motivation for insulin manipulation here might be qualified as evading weight gain instead of inducing weight loss, the two are intimately associated and sometimes cannot be effectively parsed either psychologically or physiologically.

References:
1.) 32.) Rodin G, Daneman D. Eating Disorders and IDDM. A Problematic Association. *Diabetes Care* 1992; 15: 1402-412.
2.) 4.) Cantwell R, and Steel J. Screening for Eating Disorders in Diabetes Mellitus. *Journal of Psychosomatic Research* 1996; 40 : 15-20.
3.) Daneman D, Olmsted M, Rydall A, Maharaj S, Rodin G. Eating Disorders in Young Women with Type 1 Diabetes: Prevalence, Problems and Prevention. *Hormone Research* 1998; 50: 79-86.
4.) Takii M, Uchigata Y, Nozaki T, Nishikata H, Kawal K, Komaki G, Iwamoto Y, Kubok C. Classification of Type 1 Diabetic Females With Bulimia Nervosa Into Subgroups According to Purging Behavior. *Diabetes Care* 2001; 25: 1571-575.
5.) Cantwell R, and Steel J. Screening for Eating Disorders in Diabetes Mellitus. Journal of Psychosomatic Research 1996; 40 : 15-20.
6.) Jones J, Lawson M, Daneman D, Olmsted M, Rodin G. Eating Disorders in Young Adults with Insulin Dependent Diabetes Mellitus: A Cross-Sectional Study. *British Medical Journal* 2000; 320: 1563-566.
7.) Steel JM, Young RJ, Lloyd GG, and Clarke BF. Clinically apparent eating disorders in young diabetic women: associations with painful neuropathy and other complications. *British Medical Journal* 1987; 294: 859-62.
8.) Pollock-Barziv S, Davis C. Personality Factors and Disordered Eating in Young Women with Type I Diabetes Mellitus. *Psychosomatics* 2005; 46: 11-18.
9.) Hiliard JR, Hiliard PJA. Bulimia, anorexia nervosa, and diabetes: a deadly combination. *Psychiatric Clinics of North America* 1984; 7: 367-89.

10.) Friedman S., Vila G, Timsit J, Boitard C, Mouren-Simeoni MC. Eating Disorders and Insulin Dependent Diabetes Mellitus (IDDM) relationships with glycaemic control and somatic complications. *Acta Psychiatrica Scandinavica* 1998; 97: 206-12.

11.) Bryden, K, Niel A, Mayou R, Peveler R, Fairburn C, Dunger D. Eating Habits, Body Weight, and Insulin Misuse. *Diabetes Care* 1999; 22 : 1956-960.

12.) 33.) Stancin T, Link D, Reuter J. Binge Eating and Purging in Young Women with IDDM. *Diabetes Care* 1989; 12: 601-03.

13.) Rodin G, Daneman D. Eating Disorders and IDDM. A Problematic Association. *Diabetes Care* 1992; 15: 1402-412.

14.) The Diabetes Control and Complications Trial Research Group. The effect of intensive treatment of diabetes on the development and progression of long-term complications in insulin-dependent diabetes mellitus. *New England Journal of Medicine* 1993: 329:977-86.

15.) Polonsky W, Anderson B, Lohrer P, Aponte J, Jacobson A, Cole C. Insulin Omission in women with IDDM. *Diabetes Care* 1994: 1178-185.

16.) Takii, M., G. Komaki, Y. Uchigata, M. Maeda, Y. Omori, and C. Kubo. "Differences between Bulimia Nervosa and Binge-eating Disorder in Females with Type 1 Diabetes: The Important Role of Insulin Omission." *Journal of Psychosomatic Research* 47.3 1999: 221-31. Print.

17.) Goebel-Fabbri A, Fikkan J, Franko D, Pearson K, Anderson B, Weinger K. Insulin Restriction and Associated Morbidity and Mortality in Women with Type 1 Diabetes. *Diabetes Care* 2007.

18.) Pollock-Barziv S, Davis C. Personality Factors and Disordered Eating in Young Women with Type I Diabetes Mellitus. Psychosomatics 2005; 46: 11-18.

19.) Rodin G, Olmsted MP, Rydall AC. Eating disorders in young women with type 1 diabetes mellitus. Journal of Psychosomatic Research 2002; 53: 943-49.

20.) Kaminer Y, Robbins D. Insulin Misuse: A review of an overlooked psychiatric problem. *Psychosomatics* 1989: 19-24.

21.) Rodin, G., Craven J, Littlefield C, Murray M, Daneman D. Eating disorders and intentional insulin undertreatment in adolescent females with diabetes. *Psychosomatics* 1991; 32: 171-76.

22.) Burk R, Spencer M. The Prevalence of Anorexia Nervosa, Bulimia, and Induced Glycosuria in IDDM Females. *Diabetes Educator* 1989; 15: 336-41.

23.) Affenito S, Backstrand J, Welch G, Lammi-Keefe C, Rodriguez N, Adams C. Subclinical and clinical eating disorders in IDDM negatively affect metabolic control. Diabetes Care 1997; 182-84.

24.) Nielsen, Soren. "Eating Disorders in Females with Type 1 Diabetes: An Update of a Meta-analysis." *European Eating Disorders Review* 10.4 (2002): 241-54. Print.

25.) Steiner, Hans, Winnie Kwan, Tani Graham Shaffer, Shetarra Walker, Samantha Miller, Ashwini Sagar, and James Lock. "Risk and Protective Factors for Juvenile Eating Disorders." *European Child & Adolescent Psychiatry* 12.0 (2003): 38-44.

26.) Colton, P., G. Rodin, R. Bergenstal, and C. Parkin. "Eating Disorders and Diabetes: Introduction and Overview." *Diabetes Spectrum* 22.3 (2009): 138-42.

CHAPTER 3

PATHOPHYSIOLOGY:

'PEEING OUT THE COOKIE'

The thirst of diabulimia (and diabetes, for that matter) is unlike any other thirst. It is comparable to the dehydration of the desert – a panic-inducing thirst, one which lends no indication of ever being quenched. You had might as well pour gallons of liquid into the jaws of a skeleton, watch it drain through every crevice, adhering nowhere and nourishing nothing, splashing out onto the floor in the same morphology as its entrance. Forget those overdone analogies of "raging fire" or "dry as a bone" or "parchment paper." These are grossly inadequate… Try to imagine a chronically dry mouth, so desiccated that even a segment of fruit is immobilized in its chambers, where even swallowing becomes a chore. This is not distinctive, however – the cruel paradox becomes evident when you consider that water, electrolytes, juice, fluids are all readily available to extinguish the thirst. But of what use are they? I gulp them down in mindless gluttony, liter after liter after liter…and it is as if I have not drunk them at all, for in a few hours they swim merrily through my body and run out again. The taste of water, once so pure and unobtrusive, becomes repulsive, disgusting, foreign. And my mouth, it tells me to drink more, more, more, relentlessly and tyrannically…and what choice do I have but to obey?

Towards Understanding

Preface: This chapter expounds on many of the major pathophysiological processes relevant to diabulimia, and is referenced throughout the book. It is a rather technically oriented section — a background in biochemistry will aid in its understanding. We have attempted to simplify these as much as possible without discounting their inherent intricacies. However, please be reassured that familiarity with these processes is not necessary to comprehend the illness. Rather, the purpose of this chapter is to provide a synthesis of the scientific literature as it pertains to insulin omission and weight control. As such, we encourage you to treat it as an extended footnote.

Insulin is a peptide hormone critical to metabolic functioning; it regulates a panoply of biochemical processes involving carbohydrates, fat, protein, and gene transcription. As is evident in many illnesses, the dysfunction or absence of this essential molecule is devastating on a multisystemic scale, provoking both acute, long-term, and sometimes fatal metabolic derangements. Diabulimia is but one of these pathologies, whereby insulin is foregone in order to induce particular features of the deficiency.

The hallmark of Type I diabetes is destruction of pancreatic beta-cells, which constitute the body's principal apparatus for insulin production, secretion, and regulation. Beta-cells are an essential component of the islets of Langerhans, which are discrete globular cellular clusters dispersed throughout the pancreas. These islets also contain glucagon-secreting alpha-cells and somatostatin-secreting delta-cells in a high proportion. The autoimmune process culminating in destruction of the beta-cells largely spares the other islet constituents. Glucagon and somatostatin production and secretion remain for the most part unimpaired; however, for reasons to be discussed below, become dynamically imbalanced.

Under normal circumstances, insulin and glucagon function in generally antagonistic and mutually inhibitory biochemical fashions. Insulin is released in a 'fed' state under relatively low levels of strain, promotes storage of fuel, inhibits breakdown of molecules for energy, and lowers the blood sugar. Glucagon elicits virtually opposite effects: secreted in a "fasted" state under conditions of stress, it promotes oxidation of fuels, hampers the processes responsible for shelving biochemical energy, and increases the plasma glucose. Insulin directly inhibits glucagon production in pancreatic alpha-cells by suppressing transcription of glucagon's gene, and vice versa (Chart 1). In fact, salient presence of either hormone in the system is an upstream signal to halt production and release of the other. (Glucagon, under some circumstances, does at times promote insulin *secretion*.) These reciprocal interactions are crucial to the generation and perpetuation of the central diabulimia machinery.

Glucagon	Insulin
Secreted under stress, fasting, starvation	Secreted in fed state, low stress
Inhibits insulin synthesis, secretion	Inhibits glucagon synthesis, secretion
Fuel breakdown	Fuel storage
Increases blood glucose level	Decreases blood glucose level
Stimulates gluconeogenesis	Inhibits gluconeogenesis
Stimulates glycogenolysis	Stimulates glycogenesis
Stimulates fatty acid breakdown	Stimulates fatty acid synthesis
Inhibits fatty acid synthesis	Inhibits fatty acid breakdown
Promotes ketone synthesis	Inhibits ketone synthesis
Inhibits glycolysis	Promotes glycolysis
Promotes protein catabolism	Inhibits protein catabolism

Chart 1: *Comparison between the inherent roles of insulin and glucose in normal physiology.*

The immediate role for insulin in Type I diabetes is to initiate a signaling cascade culminating in translocation of the GLUT4 "portal" molecule to the cell membrane, thereby allowing glucose to enter. Initiation of this cellular cascade is impossible sans insulin in both striated muscle (cardiac and skeletal) and adipose tissue, which comprise a lion's share of the glucose-utilizing cells in the body. The blood-brain barrier, liver, neurons, and beta-cells themselves possess different dynamics and do not require insulin for glucose entry. Without insulin, major cellular compartments cannot be nourished by carbohydrate, and the glucose is forced by default to remain in the blood plasma post-digestion. Hyperglycemia rapidly ensues, as do certain compensatory mechanisms designed to rectify both the lack of immediate sustenance for essential physical functions as well as the pathological accumulation of certain metabolites. Such is the predicament in which the body finds itself following the auto-destruction of its beta-cells – the perilous state prior to diagnosis of Type I diabetes mellitus.

It is these physiological circumstances which lie at the core of diabulimia, and which the PWDb reincarnates by manipulating their prescribed exogenous insulin regimen. We will examine the pathological processes in sequence and as they progressively influence each other in the 'diabulimia sequence.' By virtue of the "opportune" physiology, each stage and component of this adverse environment potentially contributes to weight loss/control if employed in a suitable fashion. In terms of diabulimia, it is most logical to begin with the induction of pathological hypoinsulinemia, as this triggers three important hemodynamic consequences: 1.) hyperglycemia, the development of which has been described above, 2.) hyperglucagonemia, and 3.) onset of ketogenesis.

Hyperglycemia

The crude goal of hyperglycemia in the diabulimia sequence is to expunge glucose through the urine. Each gram of glucose contains roughly 4 kilocalories, and maximum elimination via this avenue is quite an efficient manner of purging recently ingested macronutrients. A majority of the wasted calories consist of glucose in the preliminary period of insulin omission – it is only after a few hours that ketonuria manifests and the patient begins to purge "fat" through the urine. Hyperglycemia is generally present throughout the course of a diabulimic episode, unlike ketonemia. (It is possible, however, to have euglycemia in tandem with ketonemia, as is sometimes present during 1.) a hasty attempt to rectify ketosis with an insulin aliquot, which will rapidly lower blood sugar but leave ketone levels temporarily unaltered, 2.) the preliminary stages of recovery after acute DKA or chronic ketosis when the blood sugar is normalized but ketones remain provisionally in circulation.)

Blood flow through the renal system – comprising 25% of cardiac output – first passes through fenestrated glomerular capillaries into a section of the kidney tubule known as Bowman's capsule. These particular capillaries are highly porous and permit selective passage of small ions/molecules such as water, sodium, and glucose while prohibiting entrance of larger proteins such as creatine and albumin. The flow rate of fluid filtered through this segment of the nephron is termed the "glomerular filtration rate" (GFR), and differs for each substance under consideration and under varying conditions. After passing through Bowman's capsule, this "filtrate" passes through the remainder of the tubule, where it is subject to a plethora of transporters, channels, gradients, and permeabilities. Each of these determine the amount of and where in the tubule (proximal, ascending/descending Loops of Henle, convoluted, distal, collecting) the different ions/molecules will either be reabsorbed back into the bloodstream or secreted into the urine.

Appropriation of glucose from the filtrate back into the the intertubular blood system occurs in the proximal tubule of the nephron, and, under normal circumstances, is completely reabsorbed. This is largely executed by a limited number of sodium-glucose cotransporters (SGLT molecules) lining this segment of the tubule. Consequently, there is a specific threshold of glucose in the filtrate above which the carriers become completely saturated and cannot transport additional glucose back into the bloodstream. As the amount of glucose entering the tubule per unit time (the "filtered load") is the product of the GFR and concentration of glucose in the plasma, the carriers will become overwhelmed more rapidly as the blood glucose increases. There are two blood glucose values crucial to this didactic, especially in light of what the PWDb hopes to actualize. The first –

180 to 200 mg/dl, delineates the point at which the sodium-glucose transporters reach an "equilibrium" or "threshold" point, and glucose begins to spill into the urine. The second – 350 mg/dl – represents the point at which the carriers become completely saturated and cannot further increase their rates of reabsorption. *Beyond* this level, the SGLT cotransporters are overwhelmed and glucose is allowed to dissipate into the tubular urine and ultimately out of the body. No carriers for the transport of glucose exist elsewhere in the nephron, neither does the body possess an innate hormonal or intersystemic mechanism to upregulate the presence of these molecules. Therefore, any glucose neglected by the proximal tubule passes through the remainder of the kidney tubule undisturbed and exits the body through the urine with no further opportunity for reclamation. (Of note, glucose is never secreted by the tubules either.)

This renal 'purging' is partially responsible for the dramatic weight loss experienced by diabetic patients *prior to diagnosis* – the 'chronic' manifestation, where the body has been hyperglycemic for an extended time before it is clinically recognized. Excess circulating glucose is not simply apportioned and shelved in another morphology – it is literally eradicated from the body, precluding any metabolic utilization. It is not difficult, then, to understand why inducing hyperglycemia is such a powerful weight control technique. As explained, the chronic version is dangerously effective, but the 'acute' manifestation is similarly striking. An example of short-term hyperglycemic renal purging is during both subjective and objective bingeing episodes in which the patient feels a desperate urge to absolve themselves of excess caloric ingestion. They restrict the insulin otherwise dosed for the corresponding intake, and in terms of what we have discussed above, the plasma glucose level rises rapidly as it cannot be attenuated by insulin-mediated striated muscle/adipocyte absorption. The blood passes through the glomerular capillaries continuously, rendering a filtrate that is highly concentrated in glucose. This filtrate continues to the proximal tubule, where the abnormally high sugar load occupies, saturates, and completely inundates the sodium-glucose transporters, leaving a vast majority of the sugar to spill over into the urine. This entire sequence of events can be accomplished in as little as two hours, and continues for as long as the hyperglycemia is maintained. Reabsorbed glucose enters the bloodstream, which again passes through the renal filtration system, creating an iterative cycle of purging.

The thirst induced by diabulimia/diabetes serves as a compensatory mechanism designed not only to increase depleted extracellular fluid reservoirs but also to mitigate the amount of glucose lost through the urine. Polydipsia transiently increases the plasma volume (very little, as plasma is only about 8% of total bodily fluid) which slightly dilutes the blood glucose concentration. Consequently, the filtered load delivered to the nephron (GFR multiplied by the plasma concentration, ie amount per time interval) is marginally decreased. The SGLT carriers then have improved capability to scavenge glucose and the proportion relinquished to the urine decreases. Unfortunately, this effect is only temporary, as the same and subsequent cycles through the nephron induce gross osmotic diuresis sourcing from the elevated tubular fluid glucose concentration. Because the reabsorption of water is so dramatically inhibited, the plasma fluid eventually contracts and the concentration of glucose rises again, all culminating in greater urinary losses.

Hyperglucagonemia

Hyperglucagonemia is a unique feature of hypoinsulinemia as it is not considered a prerequisite for hyperglycemia nor ketogenesis, but has been demonstrated to abet the development and protraction of both processes. As mentioned, insulin and glucagon operate in a feedback system so as to maintain normal blood levels – absence of one induces action of the other. The prominent absence of insulin thus lends the effects of glucagon dominance over metabolic processes *despite* the elevated presence of glucose in the bloodstream. Through stimulation of gluconeogenesis and glycogenolysis in the liver, glucagon further exacerbates hyperglycemia and acutely underscores the visceral inability to sense an immediate availability of glucose.

During a typical day in a typical individual, pancreatic alpha-cells release a miniscule basal level of glucagon in order to protect from hypoglycemia during the interims between meals when the concentration of circulating insulin is low and the blood sugar trends downwards from the temporary lack of dietary supplementation. Although this glucogenic mechanism was designed to shield the average individual from hypoglycemic excursions, it has problematic ramifications for the diabetes/diabulimia patient. Despite euglycemia in these individuals, the alpha-cells are not presented with the inhibitory signal from circulating insulin, and therefore maintain their steady release of glucagon. (Such is one of the reasons underlying prescribing Type I diabetic patients a "basal" or continuous insulin infusion – it antagonizes this process, thereby preventing insidious blood sugar elevations.) The hormonal cluster within the islets of Langerhans is a highly sensitive interregulatory system, and endogenous derangement of one component (here, insulin) inevitably spells dysfunction of the others (glucagon and somatostatin).

Although certainly deleterious to a patient seeking to improve their diabetes control, this escalation of plasma glucagon and consequent aggravation of hyperglycemia is ideal for the purposes of the PWDb. Glucagon, as described below, also plays an ancillary role in lipolysis and ketogenesis. It is indeed the diabulimic 'dark horse,' operating in stealth but powerfully destructive. When combined with the decrease in requisite insulin and compounding of all aforementioned factors, hyperglucagonemia drives the body much closer to the potent weight-loss conditions present during the pre-diagnosis period. This lends the patient a hazardous level of control over their own metabolic furnace, a power which, given their psychological frameworks, they are guaranteed to abuse.

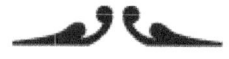

<u>Lipolysis</u>

Unfortunately, hyperglycemia (and the consequent renal removal of glucose) is not the only apparatus mobilized by the hypoinsulinemic status induced during diabulimia. When the body cannot harvest glucose from the bloodstream for metabolic consumption, it commences oxidation of both immediate dietary fat intake as well as its previously synthesized triglyceride caches. Triglyceride use is usually a normal physiological process, and does not result in disproportionate ketone production as witnessed in the pre-diagnosis or diabulimic state.

There are two metabolic centers relevant to this discussion: the striated muscle (cardiac and skeletal)/adipocytic cells, and the liver. We will begin by describing the processes specific to the former group, as these are the tissues requiring insulin for glucose ingression; liver hepatocytes *do not.*

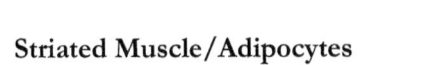

Striated Muscle/Adipocytes

Normal circumstances: In a body appropriately equipped with all insulin accoutrements, glucose enters the muscle/adipocyte cell, where it is harnessed as a first-line source of energy (prior to utilization of fatty acids for the same purpose) by processing though glycolysis. Glycolysis furnishes two molecules of pyruvate, which are then transformed by the enzyme pyruvate dehydrogenase into a molecule known as acetyl coenzyme A (acetyl CoA). Acetyl CoA enters the Krebs cycle and the oxidative phosphorylation system to produce adenosine triphosphate (ATP). ATP is the primary cellular metabolic substrate – the micromolecular equivalent of the word "energy." Whenever the amount of glucose entering these cells is in excess of their energy requirements, it is consequently shuttled towards production of triglycerides. Fatty acid synthesis in non-hepatocytes commences with conversion of the acetyl CoA derived from surplus glucose into malonyl CoA by the enzyme acetyl CoA carboxylase. This reaction represents the rate-limiting, committed step for synthesis of the fatty acid. Malonyl CoA then undergoes a series of sequential condensation reactions with more acetyl CoA molecules (derived from glucose as well) to produce a triglyceride chain of specific length. (Figure 1).

Towards Understanding

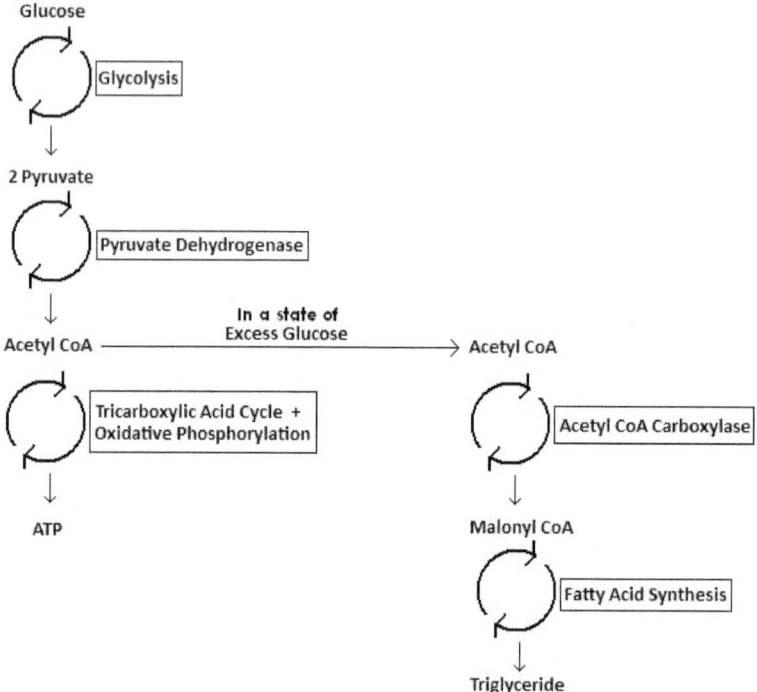

Figure 1: *Schematic of glucose pathway partitioning. The boxed terms indicate processes or specific enzymes, and terms without boxes are substrates.*

Pathologic circumstances: When glucose is unable to enter the striated/adipose cell, the above metabolic processes (ATP production, lipid synthesis) obviously cannot occur at an appreciable rate using this substrate. Hence, the balance shifts diametrically to the breakdown – instead of synthesis –of triglycerides. This process is stimulated both 1.) indirectly, by the absence of insulin, and 2.) directly, by the concomitant hormonal cascade initiated by amplified secretion of glucagon. These conditions are present both non-pathologically (i.e. during a 'fasted' state), as well as pathologically (diabulimia and poorly controlled diabetes).

Triglycerides are oxidized – usually secondary to glucose – in a variety of cells, although each differs in its profile of ability, tendency, and efficiency to utilize them as fuels. Long-chain fatty acids are first activated to fatty acyl CoAs, which cannot passively diffuse into the mitochondria. The sequential dehydrogenation, hydrolysis, and oxidation of lipid chains is executed inside this organelle; the cell must possess a scheme for conveying the lipid CoA derivatives across both mitochondrial membranes. The 'carnitine shuttle' located in the outer mitochondrial membrane surmounts this problem, granting lipid molecules access to the mitochondrial matrix. The shuttle consists of a translocase molecule (carnitine palmitoyltransferase I, aka CPT I), and CPT II.

CPT I is a crucial regulatory molecule in the sequence of fatty acid oxidation, as it controls the rate of substrate entry and therefore the yield of the reaction. Of particular importance is the fact that it is powerfully inhibited by an intermediate of fatty acid *synthesis*: malonyl CoA. This governance is important for the holistic prevention of futile cycling between breakdown and synthesis of lipids in the same cell. It is also important in the discourse regarding diabulimia – sans insulin, the striated/adipose cell possesses no excess glucose, no acetyl CoA, and consequently is devoid of malonyl CoA. Without this molecule to chaperone its activity, CPT I has free reign and lipolysis proceeds unimpeded.

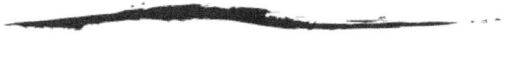

Liver

The above discussion has largely been relevant to striated muscle and adipocytes, which require insulin for glucose entry via the GLUT4 molecule. However, the dynamics of lipolysis are unique in the liver, and these are essential to understand especially in terms of their influence on ketone production (a process taking place only in liver stroma and the kidney cortex). The liver expresses a different transmembrane glucose transporter – GLUT2 – which has a high affinity for glucose. GLUT2 permits glucose access into the cytosol of the hepatocyte until equilibrium concentrations across the cell membrane are achieved. This process of ingression does *not* require insulin, and consequently liver glucose levels are hazardously elevated in diabulimia.

Given this situation, it is logical to ask why, if the liver accumulates such high amounts of glucose due to GLUT2 receptor biokinetics (in contrast to GLUT4, which under the same conditions would not permit *any* entry of glucose) that the liver would commence catabolism instead of synthesis of lipids and glycogen. We will again examine this under normal and pathological circumstances. Under normal circumstances, excess glucose translates to storage of fuel instead of breakdown. This energy shelving occurs along two synthetic pathways: 1.) glycogen production and 2.) fatty acid genesis.

- *Normal Circumstances*

The series of reactions culminating in a glycogen polymer (executed to a minor extent in muscle cells but expansively in liver) involves phosphorylation and uridylylation of glucose, which is then added sequentially to a preformed glycogen template by an enzyme known as glycogen synthase. This constitutes the rate-limiting step in glycogen synthesis; this protein is indirectly inhibited by glucagon, and, by the same token, activated by insulin. Fatty acid synthesis in hepatocytes commences with the creation of acetyl CoA through glycolysis and the catalytic actions of pyruvate dehydrogenase, similar to the processes undertaken in striated/adipose cells. Acetyl CoA is carboxylated to malonyl CoA, and shuttled towards the condensation reactions concluding in long-chain fatty acids. These lipids are packaged by the liver into primarily very-low-density-lipoproteins (VLDL) and delivered to the bloodstream

But the original paradox remains: why are these mechanisms fettered during the insulin restriction of diabulimia? The requisite substrates for both series of reactions, specifically glucose (for glycogen synthesis), and acetyl CoA (for fatty acid synthesis) should be present in disproportionately elevated amounts due to profligate hyperglycemic mechanisms. Glucose can enter unimpeded through GLUT2, so where and how, then, does the obligate monkey wrench operate? The answer lies in the severe disturbance of glucagon levels secondary to and perpetuated by chronic hypoinsulinemia.

- *Pathologic circumstances*

First, the presence (and obviously, upregulation) of glucagon levels leads to phosphorylation and consequent inhibition of glycogen synthase (which, as described above, catalyzes the limiting step in glycogen formation), despite excessive levels of available glucose.[4]

The biochemical curtailing of triglyceride synthesis is highly complex, but the crux lies in the regulation of glycolysis and pyruvate conversion. This surveillance inhibits formation of acetyl CoA itself, as the body shuts down the systems generating this crucial constituent of fatty acid elongation from the onset. This is accomplished by myriad multiple regulatory sites of glycolysis in the liver that are potentially affected by glucagon's hormonal actions.

> ➤ The first is glucokinase, the liver-specific isozyme of hexokinase, which catalyzes the first committed phosphorylation in glycolysis. The intracellular hepatocyte machinery senses an upward trend in blood sugar through this enzyme, which then phosphorylates cytosolic glucose molecules and dedicates them to the glycolytic pathway. This cellular apparatus effectively lowers/maintains the plasma glucose level. Panreatic islets aid the process by sensing the increase in blood sugar, releasing insulin, and inhibiting the secretion of glucagon. In the pre-diagnosis stage, poorly controlled diabetes, and diabulimia, this entire "hepatic glucose sensor" is sabotaged. The presence of elevated glucagon downregulates the transcription of glucokinase, ensuring that the blood sugar remains elevated while simultaneously inhibiting the formation of pyruvate and ultimately acetyl CoA.[8]

> ➤ The next hepatic regulatory site for glycolysis is 6-phosphofructo-1-kinase, which converts fructose 6-phophate into fructose-1,6-bisphosphate in the committed step of hepatic glycolysis. Through its complex biodynamic actions on the secondary regulator fructose-2,6-bisphosphate, glucagon inhibits the formation of fructose-1,6-bisphosphate and derails further steps in glycolysis.

> ➤ The absence of both fructose-1,6-bisphophate and insulin further dampen the activity of pyruvate kinase, a downstream enzyme in glycolysis catalyzing the irreversible conversion of phosphoenolpyruvate into pyruvate.

> ➤ Pyruvate dehydrogenase is the last enzyme involved in the overall conversion of glucose into acetyl CoA. It is an essential regulatory site of carbohydrate metabolism, as it directly precedes entry into the tricarboxylic acid (Krebs) cycle. Pyruvate dehydrogenase is inhibited by glucagon (and conversely, activated by insulin), resulting in low levels of acetyl CoA *originating from glucose*. It will

become important further in the chapter to differentiate the provenance of acetyl CoA (especially in regard to the genesis of ketone bodies) – which can source from the glycolytic pathway described above, or mechanisms of lipolysis.

All of these mechanisms operate in concert to decrease the cellular concentration of pyruvate, but glucagon's effects are not exhausted here.

The reigning scientific consensus maintains that an elevated glucagon:insulin proportion switches the liver from a lipogenic to a lipolytic/ketogenic profile (rather than absolute amounts of either hormone). This is the first requirement for initiation of ketone synthesis. However, the increased hormonal ratio is inadequate to actualize the production of ketone bodies; this is stimulated by the magnitude of insulin absence. The degree of insulin deficiency determines the rate and quantity of fat mobilization from the body's reservoirs to the liver, where they can be oxidized and transformed into ketone bodies. Interstitial adipocytes are the earliest recruits, but advanced insulin deficiency can damage other fat-dense cell types such as supportive Schwann cells and oligodendrocytes in the peripheral and central nervous systems, respectively. (Hormone-sensitive lipase, the enzyme responsible for catalyzing the hydrolysis of stored triacylglycerols, is the primary effector of somatic fatty acid marshaling. Insulin, in a nutritionally satiated state, dephosphorylates a serine residue on this protein and thereby inhibits its hydrolytic activity. Without insulin, hormone-sensitive lipase is activated through unimpeded efforts of other fast-acting lipolytic hormones, driving the release of free fatty acids to the liver.[3]) Contrary to the prerequisite for absolute insulin deficiency, scientists have demonstrated that an absolute glucagon excess is not required for the development of ketosis, although it abets the process as illustrated by early experiments on pancreatectomized patients.

Levels of other substances counter-regulating insulin are also intimately involved in the pathogenesis of DKA, although to a lesser extent than that of glucagon. These include primarily molecules involved in the physiological response to stress and inflammation and their liberation is abetted by abnormal insulin-deficient states. Hyperglycemia also triggers a pro-inflammatory state rendering the body prone to the unwarranted autogeneration of cytokines, reactive oxygen species, and steroidal imbalances, not dissimilar to those processes inducing the long-term complications outlined in Chapter 5. The hormones implicated in DKA include cortisol, estrogen, and catecholamines; inflammatory markers of note are TNF-alpha, IL-6 and IL-8.[9]

Ketogenesis

Ketone bodies are produced in the mitochondrial matrices of hepatocytes and kidney cortex, where, conveniently, fats are also oxidized to produce the acetyl CoA molecules from which they are derived. These acetyl CoAs are prevented from integrating into fatty acid *synthesis* by the high levels of glucagon, which induce lipolysis in the first place. They also inhibit acetyl CoA carboxylase from converting acetyl CoA to malonyl CoA (which leads to lipo*genesis*) in a futile cycle. It is easy to misconceive that the acetyl CoA derived from the glycolytic/pyruvate dehydrogenase pathway might also be used to create ketone bodies. However, the fact that glycolysis came to fruition implies the existence of a high insulin:glucagon ratio, directly opposite to that encountered in the ketogenic state (which produces acetyl CoA from the degradation of *triglycerides*). In gross essence, the two circumstances are mutually exclusive: ketogenesis requires a high glucagon:insulin ratio, whereas glycolysis requires a high insulin:glucagon ratio. Therefore, the acetyl CoA produced from one pathway cannot insert into the other because the singular environment of the cell/organ prohibits it. This is why it is technically inaccurate and simplistic to say that "hyperglycemia makes ketones" – there are many intermediary mechanisms in operation. High blood sugar certainly does contribute to ketone formation through the glucagon:insulin ratio subversion. However, when exogenous insulin (which is more powerful than endogenous glucagon) is thrown into the melee, this process is dramatically reduced or even eradicated, *even in the presence of hyperglycemia.*

To illustrate this point, consider the following scenario (which does not necessarily have to be specific to diabulimia): A patient eats a certain portion of food, and gives herself a certain dose of insulin. However, whether advertently or inadvertently, this dose of insulin is inadequate to cover the carbohydrates present in what she has consumed. Her blood sugar rises, perhaps even over 400 mg/dl, but *there will be minimal ketone formation* for the next few hours due to the presence of circulating insulin, which inhibits both the formation of glucagon as well as a majority of the processes resulting in ketonemia.

- ***Normal and Pathologic Circumstances***

Ketogenesis is initiated by the condensation of two acetyl CoA molecules to form acetoacetyl CoA, followed by further condensation of acetoacetyl CoA with another molecule of acetyl CoA to form HMG-CoA. The latter reaction is catalyzed by HMG-CoA synthase (similar to, but not a replica of the respective enzyme and molecule which are intermediates in cholesterol synthesis). HMG-CoA is then cleaved by HMG-CoA lyase to yield the first ketone body, acetoacetic acid (Figure 1). The regulatory mechanism for this enzyme is still to be elucidated. As such, it is unknown what dynamic drives the dramatic crescendo of ketone bodies such as that witnessed in moderate to severe DKA, but the theories are multifactorial. Primary contributing factors are the processes realized in the liver secondary to insulin deficiency, commencing with uninhibited fatty acid oxidation – a mechanism unfortunately reinforced through the ancillary dietary pathway. As the concentration of exogenous long chain fatty acids increases, the cellular concentration of malonyl CoA - inhibitor of fatty acid degradation – decreases through inhibition of acetyl CoA carboxylase. (Recall that acetyl CoA carboxylase catalyzes the formation of malonyl CoA from acetyl CoA, and is actively inhibited by long-chain fatty acids.) It follows that as more fats are ingested during the insulin deficient/hyperglycemic state of diabulimia, more fats are oxidized, levels of acetyl CoA rise, and more ketones are produced in a vicious feedback mechanism.[5] Ketone body genesis occurs at a rate far exceeding that at which the peripheral tissues are able to utilize, leading to accretion in the bloodstream and subsequent purging through the urine. This inadequate metabolic clearance is actually what scientists believe to be the driving factor underlying hyperketonemia, rather than overproduction.[6] Plasma ketone body concentrations can reach 200-300 fold the levels witnessed in normal fasting ketosis [7,10] and in one study, up to 1000.[12]

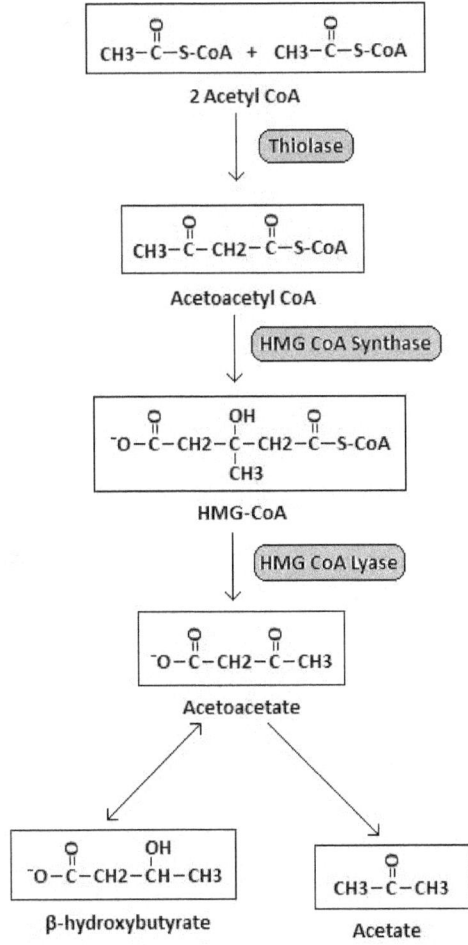

Figure 2 : *Synthesis of ketone bodies. White boxes show substrates/products, and grey ovals show enzymes.*

Acetoacetic acid is processed further into two other major ketone bodies. The first is beta-hydroxybutyric acid, which is simply the reduced form of acetoacetic acid. ('Acetoacetic acid' and 'acetoacetate' are the same core molecule, but labeled differently depending on their protonation status at different pH levels; the same applies to 'beta-hydroxybutyric acid and beta-hydroxybutyrate.') Its formation depends on the number of reducing equivalents produced through preceding lipolysis reactions. Acetoacetic acid and beta-hydroxybutyric acid are relatively strong acids that are completely deprotonated at physiological pH. When present in pathological amounts (200-300 times normal levels), these molecules completely inundate the hematological buffering systems and lead to a state of metabolic acidosis. Acetone is the other ketone body deriving from a slow decarboxylation of acetoacetic acid, and is generally only formed during conditions of severe ketoacidosis when concentrations of acetoacetic acid are perilously elevated. Acetone does not contribute to acidosis as it cannot release hydrogen ions, but the blood is so saturated with the compound under these circumstances that its odor becomes detectable in the patient's breath – the source of the "fruity, pear-like" aroma of a patient in ketoacidosis. Structural permutations of these ketone bodies are, of course, replete but individually present in fractionally minor amounts.

The enzymes necessary for ketone synthesis, namely HMG-CoA synthase and HMG-CoA lyase, are only present in liver and kidney tissue; conversely, the enzymes enabling utilization of ketones for ATP production are expressed only in other non-hepatic organs. Hence, the two systems are mutually exclusive, which ensures that the cells synthesizing ketone bodies are not biochemically equipped to oxidize them, and vice versa.

Ketones are actually efficient fuels for a number of tissues during fasting, although they are certainly not the energy of preference.[1] Glucose is by default oxidized first, followed by free fatty acids. Ketones (and *then* proteins) are the last resorts, but necessitated in the absence of other feasible fuels. They are especially important for brain function during prolonged hyperglycemia, as fats do not facilely traverse the blood-brain barrier. (In addition to glucose, the brain typically uses minor but appreciable amounts of acetoacetic acid and beta-hydroxybutyric acid on a daily basis as its primary source of nourishment. When their bloodstream concentration becomes salient, as in a PWDb with sufficiently severe insulin omission, the rate of their crossing the blood-brain barrier rises in proportion. The amount of ketone bodies utilized by the brain can accrue to such a great degree that they eventually override glucose as a source of fuel. This phenomenon explains why, in part, insulin must be reintroduced gradually during recovery so as not to shock the neural tissue with an unreasonably abrupt transition from ketone bodies back to glucose.[2] This is addressed in a later chapter.)

Acetoacetic acid and beta-hydroxybutyric acid are short organic acids which can diffuse across muscle and adipocyte cell membranes sans receptor (unlike glucose). Within the mitochondria of non-hepatic tissues, ketones are converted back to acetoacetic acid. In a reaction catalyzed by the enzyme acetoacetate:succinyl-CoA transferase (a protein markedly absent in liver parenchyma), acetoacetic acid is transformed into its CoA derivative, where it can then enter the Krebs cycle for ATP production. In this fashion, ketones efficiently replace glucose as a medium of nourishment for a majority of tissues.

Ketones are also partially responsible for the short-term "sparing" of physical muscle for the endogenous production of glucose. Over a chronic period of insulin omission, the body cannibalizes the protein present in muscle and visceral organ cells to effect gluconeogenesis due to glucagon elevation. This, however, is more of an end-stage occurrence – catabolism of muscle and visceral organ protein is the body's last resort, and ketone utilization is one of the desperate final attempts to conserve these tissues before employing such a drastic measure.[5] Although rarely measured in a clinical setting, elevated levels of these serum amino acids usually indicates a highly advanced/sustained stage of metabolic abnormality, as the irreversible breakdown of proteins represents the ultimate compensatory effort in a sequence of available fuels, beginning with glucose, continuing with fats, and followed by ketones. Although there is always a baseline level of muscle breakdown during states of insulin deficiency, it does not usually manifest significantly until very severe degrees

---

5   It must be emphasized here that ketone formation is actually a profoundly physiological compensation for certain non-adverse circumstances such as fasting or low-carbohydrate diets. In such cases, moderately elevated ketone levels are nontoxic and actually necessary for survival, as they represent the only appreciable source of utilizable cellular fuel. Also, no studies have conclusively proven that ketones by themselves cause end-organ or vascular damage, compared to the advanced-glycosylation end products (AGEs) generated as a consequence of chronic hyperglycemia. This is to say that the "complication" stigma associated with diabetic ketosis places a great deal of blame for organ damage on the ketones themselves, when it is actually the insulin deficiency and consequent hyperglycemia that are the root of the destruction. In the theoretical absence of hyperglycemia, isolated hyperketonemia would be relatively less damaging.

of DKA are attained. Most of the weight loss during early stages, apart from water, entails partitioning of fat – channeling directly into the psychological motivation of omitting insulin. When these adverse conditions persist, the body begins to attack its own muscle so as to sustain the demands of both 1.) gluconeogenesis even in the face of hyperglycemia – due to high circulating plasma glucagon, and 2.) energy production.

The metabolic pathways of each amino acid towards ATP genesis is unique, and here we will only highlight a few. There is a specific subset that can be converted to solely ketones (leucine and lysine), others to both glucose and ketones (isoleucine, phenylalanine, tryptophan, tyrosine, and threonine), and a third group to only glucose (all save for leucine, lysine, and the glucogenic/ketogenic amino acids). The ways by which glucose and ketones produce ATP have been discussed previously. Some, such as valine and isoleucine, ultimately undergo transformation into succinyl CoA through intermediates such as propionyl CoA and methylmalonyl CoA, which enters directly into the Krebs cycle for energy production. (Referring back to the 'larger picture,' this phenomenon explains why PWDbs manage to retain some of their muscle tissue during the initial phases of the illness, albeit with palpable loss; the body spares these tissues until the final phases.

In the ketoacidotic state created by the PWDb, the production of ketones far exceeds that which is required for use by the tissues. Consequently, there is renal purging of these molecules, similar to that described previously for hyperglycemia. In fact, clinicians rely on this mechanism of urinary clearance during periods of ketoacidosis to eliminate or at least attenuate their abnormal accumulation. (This is accomplished using a low-rate infusion 'insulin drip' to antagonize the ketone-producing machinery as described above, enabling the kidney to gradually excrete them. Respiratory clearance through acid-CO_2 buffering is feasible neither in terms of rate nor energy expenditure.) Renal elimination of ketone bodies also helps to compensate for the metabolic acidosis. As diabulimia and undiagnosed diabetes progress, the osmotic diuresis induced by hyperglycemia incrementally exacerbates dehydration, which likewise progressively compromises renal function. The kidneys ultimately reach a point of (temporary and reversible) prerenal failure, and can no longer as efficiently rid the body of ketones, which accumulate in the bloodstream. When the plasma concentration of ketones reaches a certain threshold, the patient becomes fully decompensated. They are no longer able to cope autonomously with the physiological derangements, leading to clinical presentation.

Unlike the renal physiology involving glucose, there is no evidence to support a 'transport maximum' tubular reabsorption rate for the major ketones (acetoacetic acid and 3-hydroxybutyrate), even in juvenile diabetics prior to insulin treatment. They are not bound to plasma proteins and are therefore ultrafilterable; their 'filtered load' is equal to the glomerular filtration rate multiplied by the plasma concentration. Below certain filtered loads, ie 'thresholds,' acetoacetic acid and beta-hydroxybutyric acid are completely reabsorbed.[14] As mentioned above, hyperketonemia is theorized to result from the compounding of both 1.) elevated ketone production due to lack of insulin and increased levels of circulating triglycerides mobilized from adipose stores and dietary intake 2.) plateaued/decreased ability for peripheral utilization (tissue removal capacities become saturated as the plasma concentration is amplified).[12] The plasma ketone concentration and glomerular filtered load rise in proportion. Above those particular thresholds, ketones spill over into the tubular fluid, but the kidney still expends effort to reabsorb them. Ketone reabsorption rates increase in a linear relationship with the filtered load during starvation.[15] Thus, there is a threshold, but no transport maximum for ketones. Considering this renal biodynamic, some have hypothesized that a majority of the renal purging of ketones is instead attributed to tubular secretion, induced by the toxic levels attained during ketoacidosis. Also interesting to note is the fact that excretory rates in juvenile diabetics not receiving insulin treatment (theoretically similar to diabulimia patients) was augmented by 28% compared to controls with similar levels of infused ketones.[11]

Diabulimia therefore has two 'purging' mechanisms through manipulation of renal physiology: the loss of glucose as glycosuria, and the loss of fat/proteins as ketonuria. Patients are essentially urinating food – which is obviously highly convenient as a purging mechanism. Indeed, it is far more efficacious than diuretics or laxatives, which do little but to excrete filtered water/ions/stool which have already been excoriated of any nutrients or calories, and would have been eliminated anyway. (Only drugs like orlistat, which literally prevents reabsorption of fat in the intestine, truly 'purge' calories.) The lack of insulin in a pre-diagnosed diabetic/diabulimic patient literally induces "peeing away calories," not to mention the concomitant loss of electrolytes and fluids similar to that produced by diuretics and enemas.

However, like other common purging mechanisms (e.g. vomiting, excessive exercise), complete restriction of insulin is not a vacuum or 'true starvation' state. Namely, not all calories are purged – glucose and ketones are reabsorbed and rendered usable by the tissues for at least a baseline survival level. The resulting distended pool of metabolites remains in the body until they can be excreted in the urine (glucose and ketones) or exhaled (ketones). Until then, they are still utilizable by the tissues – the limiting factor is the tissues and their intrinsic circumstantial capacities. Therefore, some of the food ingested translates into stored calories if consumed in excess of a daily caloric limit, *despite the lack of insulin*. Glucose is the only macronutrient that requires insulin for uptake, but other molecules, such as fat and protein, have their own specific non-insulin-dependent receptors promoting cellular uptake from the bloodstream. Although the chronic absence of insulin will powerfully induce breakdown of other macronutrients through the mechanisms described in this chapter (which for the most part overrides their use by peripheral tissues), it does not do so comprehensively. Ingestion of fat or protein with an acute rather than chronic deficiency of insulin will not effect the same purging, and a higher proportion of the calories from these non-glucose macronutrients can be metabolized, due to their insulin-*independent* properties. A few ketones might form, some glucose might spill over into the urine, some endogenous proteins might be catabolized due to the transiently increased glucagon:insulin ratio, but a reasonable fraction is rendered usable. This is why some *bingeing* PWDbs present with a history of cyclical weight gain instead of holistic loss. *Restrictive* PWDbs, on the other hand, do not have a reservoir of ingested calories – the only source of energy that their body feasibly uses is dismantling of its own tissues. This actually leads to holistic weight loss in the circumstances of *both* acute and chronic insulin deficiency.

References:

1.) Balassed, E. O., F. Fery, and M. A. Neef. "Changes Induced by Exercise in Rates of Turnover and Oxidation of Ketone Bodies in Fasting Man." Journal of Applied Physiology 44.1 (1978): 5-11. Print.

2.) Daniel, P.M., E.R. Love, S.R. Moorehouse, O.E. Pratt, and Penelope Wilson. "Factors Influencing Utilisation of Ketone-bodies by Brain in Normal Rats and Rats with Ketoacidosis." The Lancet 298.7725 (1971): 637-38.

3.) Stralfors, P., Bjorgrell, P., Bellfrage, P. "Hormonal Regulation of Hormone-Sensitive Lipase in Intact Adipocytes: Identification of Phosphorylated Sites and Effects on the Phosphorylation by Lipolytic Hormones and Insulin." Proceedings of the National Academy of Sciences 81.11 (1984): 3317-321.

4.) Jiang, G., and B. Zhang. "Glucagon and Regulation of Glucose Metabolism." American Journal of Physiology - Endocrinology and Metabolism 284 (2003).

5.) McGarry, J. D., and D. W. Foster. "Regulation of Hepatic Fatty Acid Oxidation and Ketone Body Production." Annual Review of Biochemistry 49 (1980): 395-420.

6.) Owen, O., BSB Block, M. Patel, G. Boden, M. McDonough, T. Kreulen, CR Shuman, and GA Reichard. "Human Splanchnic Metabolism during Diabetic Ketoacidosis."Metabolism 26.4 (1977): 381-98.

7.) Devlin, Thomas M. Textbook of Biochemistry with Clinical Correlations. Hoboken, N.J: J. Wiley, 2006. Print.

8.) Iynedjian, P., D. Jotterand, T. Nouspikel, M. Asfari, and PR Pilot. "Transcriptional Induction of Glucokinase Gene by Insulin in Cultured Liver Cells and Its Repression by the Glucagon-CAMP System." Journal of Biological Chemistry 264.36 (1989).

9.) Stentz FB, Umpierrez GE, Cuervo R, Kitabchi AE. Proinflammatory cytokines, markers of cardiovascular risks, oxidative stress, and lipid peroxidation in patients with hyperglycemic crises. Diabetes 2004; 53:2079.

10.) Laffel, L. Ketone bodies: a review of physiology, pathophysiology and application of monitoring to diabetes. Diabetes/Metabolism Reviews Rev 1999; 15: 412-426

11.) Wildenhoff, K. E. "Tubular Reabsorption and Urinary Excretion of Acetoacetate and 3-Hydroxybutyrate in Normal Subjects and Juvenile Diabetics." Acta Medica Scandinavica 201 (1977): 63-67.

12.) Keller, U., M. Lustenberger, J. Muller-Brand, PPPG Gerber, and W. Stauffacher. "Human Ketone Body Production and Utilization Studied Using Tracer Techniques: Regulation by Free Fatty Acids, Insulin, Catecholamines, and Thyroid Hormones."Diabetes/Metabolism Reviews 5.3 (1989): 285-98.

13.) Fery, F., and E. O. Balasse. "Ketone Body Production and Disposal in Diabetic Ketosis. A Comparison with Fasting Ketosis." Diabetes 34.4 (1985): 326-32.

14.) Sapir, D.G., and O.E. Owen. "Renal Conservation of Ketone Bodies during Starvation."Metabolism 24.1 (1975): 23-33.

15.) Martin, Helen Eastman, and Arne N. Wick. "Quantitative Relationships Between Blood And Urine Ketone Levels In Diabetic Ketosis." Journal of Clinical Investigation 22.2 (1943): 235-41.

16.) Balasse EO, Fery F. Ketone body production and disposal: effects of fasting, diabetes, and exercise. Diabetes/Metabolism Reviews 1989; 5: 247-270.

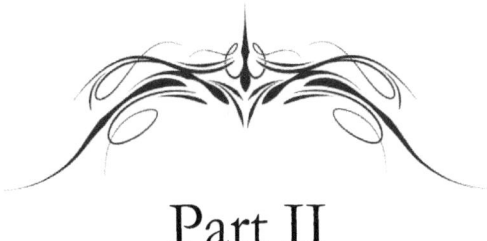

Part II

TOWARDS RECOGNITION

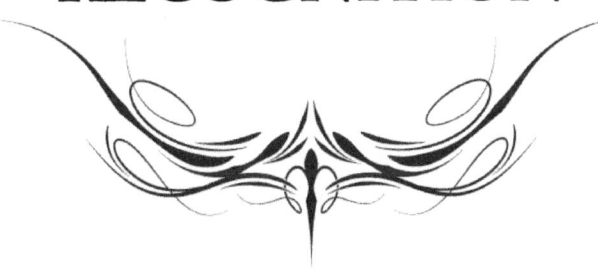

CHAPTER 4

CHARACTERISTICS

There were times when I realized I absolutely needed an iota of insulin. Those mornings I would drag myself out of bed, heart pounding, mouth crusted with dehydrated saliva, and grab a syringe from the forsaken box at the bottom of my desk drawer. The process of waking up in itself was an ordeal, the most acute torture of the day – surviving the remainder became feasible after that A.M. litmus test. Nighttime, on the other hand, was a study in interruptions: trudging four or five times to the bathroom to urinate and at other points just to gulp down copious amounts of water. Sometimes the breathing did it – the gasping for nourishment, some inner impetus that prompted a greedy, insatiable ingestion of air. It suffocated, simultaneously it deprived. Other times it was the thirst, or the stomachaches, or the physical exhaustion. Those days, those mornings – those were the limit, the breaking point even for the seemingly invincible determination I had quietly nurtured.

Omitting insulin was to negotiate a precarious balance between flaccid dysfunction and barely being able to accomplish the day's tasks. Just one dose, *I promised, glaring with malicious ambivalence at the needle I held in my hand, scarcely mustering the strength to plunge it into my dry skin.* You're living on borrowed time, anyway…

A few hours later, I would lie on my bed, momentarily relieved from thirst or rapid breathing or fast heartbeats or stomach aches. I love insulin, I thought, smiling ironically, as I once again disconnected and decommissioned my pump for the next few hours or days or weeks. I couldn't even gather the energy to shed a tear.

Towards Recognition

This chapter is intended to enumerate and describe the presenting "characteristics" of diabulimia patients. We have divided it into five overall sections:

1.) *Insulin Manipulation Patterns*
2.) *Epidemiology*
3.) *Case Descriptions*
4.) *Symptoms*
5.) *The Clinical Appointment*
6.) *Laboratory Values*

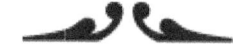

Insulin Manipulation Patterns

When discussing insulin omission, especially clinically, it is useful to know exactly *how* the patient executes this purging. The theoretical "Cartesian plot" of insulin omission has three dimensions: frequency, amplitude, and duration. Frequency signifies how often an insulin dose is omitted or reduced. Amplitude signifies how much of the insulin is foregone – this can range from completely eliminating a dose or only dampening its value. (For this variable, insulin "restriction" can be considered semantically distinct from insulin "omission," but in all other settings the two terms are used interchangeably.) Duration signifies the longitudinal extent of time for which the adverse behaviors concerning insulin have been executed. (The case of an insulin pump further complicates matters as it includes multiple "basal" rates, infused as a short-acting insulin such as Novolog or Humalog during the day in a constant or intermittent pattern. A patient might have a basal rate of 1 unit/hour for the entire day, or 0.5 units/hour from 9am-5pm, no basal from 5-9pm, and 1.4 unit/hr the rest of the day, etc. This basal rate, here for the purpose of clarity, can be considered as an insulin "dose." It is manipulated in the same way – the technical aspects are only slightly different.)

Each insulin dose for the PWDb can vary on all three parameters, although sometimes the patient develops a particular pattern. This introduces a fourth variable: consistency, namely, the degree of reproducibility of each of first three. If this theoretical component of consistency held an analogous counterpart in the real world, the clinician's duties would be dramatically simplified. Unfortunately, the considerable variation in insulin omission patterns – other compensatory behaviors notwithstanding – renders diabulimia frustratingly unpredictable. Patients vacillate between drastically different sets of frequency, amplitude, and duration, sometimes with intermittent periods of total/nominative compliance. (For example, a patient might fail to dose for 'snacks' but gives full insulin for what they consider to be 'meals' on one day; following this, they take proper amounts of insulin for a few days but the following week omit insulin completely. Such patterns might cycle or become progressively worse.) Therefore, attempting to state that a particular patient "omits x amount of insulin, y times a week, and has been doing so for z number of days/weeks/years," is not entirely pragmatic.

As explained in previous chapters, diabulimia still lacks an official clinical label, and this deficiency in the medical arsenal also entails a salient lack of criteria for diagnosis. Some will argue that if insulin omission is considered an inappropriate compensatory behavior (ICB) in bulimia nervosa (purging subtype) and anorexia nervosa (both restrictive and binge-eating/purging subtypes), it can subsequently be quantified and defined according to DSM criteria. However, the permutations of insulin omission patterns complicate this assessment, and studies must yet be conducted in order to determine what parameters of omission are associated with statistically significant outcomes. Subjects might completely deprive their bodies of insulin for weeks to months on end, or perpetually underdose themselves. Combinations are numerous, ranging from short to protracted intervals, and the spectrum of dosage is similarly diverse. In various studies, women report that patterns of insulin omission range from "occasionally" and "rarely" to "always" for a given period of time.[6,7] Some researchers have defined severe insulin omission as an ICB to be the curtailing of more than 25% of a patient's prescribed daily dosage.[5]

Others will argue that the entire discussion of quantification is moot, as intentionally foregoing even an iota of insulin for weight control is pathological. It qualifies as what is generally referred to as 'Eating Disorder Not Otherwise Specified (EDNOS),' which tragically in most clinical circumstances is either misrecognized, ignored, or undertreated with a 'watch-and-wait' approach. Ideally, this condition should immediately be addressed, especially as 1.) EDNOS patients frequently progress to full-threshold eating disorders without treatment, 2.) therapy is similar to that of bulimia and/or anorexia nervosas, and 3.) early intervention even in these subthreshold patients is associated with reduced morbidity and mortality.[21]

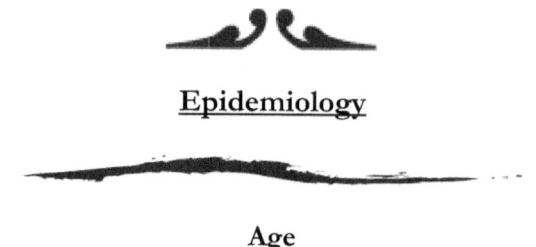

Epidemiology

Age

Although diabulimia can present at virtually any age, the greatest percentage of PWDbs is in the demographic under thirty.[7] Studies incorporating insulin-dependent diabetic females of widely disparate ages demonstrate a singular pattern: insulin omission was initiated during adolescent years and, in extreme cases, perpetuated through adulthood.[8, 9] Although diabulimia is not incident/prevalent in pre-adolescents, its incidence rises dramatically following pubertal onset. For example, in a study originally involving pre-adolescent females (conducted by Bryden et al., 1994), the number of patients admitting to insulin omission only became significant after an eight-year follow-up when the subjects were well into their teenage years.[14] In terms of cognitive development and maturity, younger adolescents usually mentate concretely, i.e. they cannot abstract consequences longitudinally. Material entities (such as weight, clothes, appearance, food, and freedom) adopt more importance than intangible concepts such as long-term health, complications from poorly controlled diabetes, and the like. In general, metabolic control is reported to be worst during teenage years even in the absence of eating anomalies, which might cause the intentional insulin omission practices in this demographic.[10-12]

Of note, there are reports of postpartum insulin omission for the purpose of controlling gestational weight gain. This might present as diabulimia *de novo*, or as residual from a previous bout of the illness. Women are – more often than not – internally motivated to manage glycemic levels antepartum to prevent fetal glucotoxicity.

Due to both the increase in eating disorder incidence as well as accessibility of common triggers/motivations of diabulimia in recent years, the prevalence of pre- and post-adolescent PWDbs has also been amplified. Not uncommonly, clinicians treat patients in their late 20's or mid-thirties who have either recently developed diabulimia or have suffered from the illness since adolescence. (The latter exemplifies the "overlap" effect of current diabulimia statistics, in which the *prevalence* of diabulimia incorrectly causes a statistical increase in the *incidence* by representation/calculation in different populations). Analogously, the incidence of pre-pubescent patients presenting with symptoms characteristic of diabulimia has been higher in recent years (anecdotal evidence).

Theories addressing the specificity of this demographic abound, but clinical consensus reveals that the numerous psychological stressors which arise and accrue during adolescence contribute largely to both insulin-omitting and non-insulin-omitting eating disorders. This includes changes in body morphology, peer pressure to emulate cultural icons, increased dietary freedom, heightened sense of independence, entitlement to rebel against authority, teenage "angst," among myriad others. This is also the age when many Type I patients are diagnosed with diabetes; superimposing the stressors of the illness (such as food control, weight gain, and dampened social spontaneity) on an already volatile interval of life leaves these particular patients perilously exposed to psychiatric problems like diabulimia.

Gender

The incidence of eating disorders and insulin omission in type I diabetics is generally far greater in females than in males. Males consistently fail to demonstrate a greater tendency for disturbed eating behaviors (especially insulin omission) than females.[14, 15] One study reported that Type I diabetic males score higher on the 'drive for thinness' subscale within the Eating Disorder Inventory questionnaire as compared to their non-diabetic control counterparts.[22] In general, the prevalence of diabulimia follows suit with the overarching pattern of non-insulin-omitting eating disorders: in comparison to controls, males are less likely than females to intentionally misuse insulin, especially for the purpose of weight control. (This pattern, however, has shifted in recent years, but female gender is still typically regarded as a risk factor for disordered eating.)

Towards Recognition

Males are equipped with intrinsically higher and more adaptable metabolic rates, enabling them to consume more calories with a slower velocity of weight gain. This characteristic can mitigate the psychological strain of limiting polyphagic intake post-diagnosis. Many girls are also diagnosed with Type I inter-adolescence, when gender-specific physical transformations (such as breast and hip development) might exacerbate body dysmorphia.

Although a rather simplistic nuance, this sex disparity might further be explained by contemporary weight culture, in which young girls are inculcated with rail-thin female role models, whereas muscular, bulky men on the other hand feature as the ideal aesthetic. Clinicians have tentatively proposed some terms for the latter – "muscle dysmorphia" and "bigorexia."[20] Concerning weight specifically, female efforts are geared largely towards loss or maintenance rather than gain, whereas a high proportion of males exhibit a tendency towards the opposite trend (needless to say, some overlap does exist). Accruing rather than shedding muscular mass is a significant cultural fixation, and is in fact *abetted* by the presence of insulin. The hormone promotes anabolic synthesis and shelving of muscle protein, and it is fundamentally counterintuitive to cannibalize muscle secondary to insulin omission if hypertrophy is the ultimate goal.

This is not to say that males should be excluded from the putative diabulimia population. These studies have limitations [within our particular context] in that they only analyze insulin omission under the umbrella of eating disorder ICB's, which might underestimate the true prevalence of insulin omission in the male demographic. Selection of the diabetic study population for these eating disorder investigations is often biased towards patients who present with more well-recognized compensatory behaviors such as vomiting and excessive exercise, and might exclude patients who have eating disorders manifesting only with insulin omission. Anecdotally, males actually constitute an appreciable number of patients who use insulin omission for the purpose of weight control.

Miscellaneous

Race has not proved to be a major factor in the development of diabulimia, or has not been examined extensively to determine any outstanding distinctions or risk factors.

The same applies to socioeconomical status, although some clinicians have testified that patients are most frequently of middle-class background. Contrary to popular belief, diabulimia is in no way a "rich man's" or "poor man's" disease. People of all financial statuses are vulnerable to developing these patterns of behavior. To say that affluent diabetic patients have more resources with which to foster an insulin-omitting eating disorder (both monetarily and psychologically) is a crude generalization and discounts the multifaceted nature of the illness. Reducing diabulimia (or any eating disorder) to the 'leisurely ability to concern oneself with weight and eating' does both physician and patient a disservice. By the same token, postulating that lower-income patients are more susceptible to this illness because they do not have adequate resources to buy medical supplies (thus facilitating lower insulin dosing and poor diabetes management) is a grossly incorrect interpretation of diabulimia. These individuals intentionally do not take insulin out of necessity, but their psychological framework is still intact.

A logical question deriving from this discussion is whether PWDbs are more commonly encountered among patients with or without insulin pumps. Unfortunately, there is currently no clear clinical data on this issue. Theoretically, both injections/pens and insulin pumps (the two most common types of insulin administration) hold significant advantages and disadvantages for the insulin-curtailing and deceptive mechanisms necessary for diabulimia. A phenomenon likely to be encountered with either modality is the serendipitous 'discovery' of diabulimia. This commences with elimination of single/multiple shots/boluses (simply forgotten, or prompted by irritation, exhaustion, and disillusionment) *without* adverse eating or ideation concerning weight. The blood sugar consequently runs high for a few hours or a few days, the patient loses some tangible caloric/water weight, and they make the unfortunate connection between insulin deficiency and body mass. Depending on their particular baseline psyche, they are consequently 1.) cognitively untainted, continuing to allow doses to slip through the cracks as a reflection of carelessness but not weight manipulation, 2.) averse to the uncomfortable somatic symptoms of hyperglycemia, prompting a return to proper management, or 3.) made more vulnerable to omitting insulin for weight or intake control by internalizing the observation of weight loss. Injections/pens are an admittedly cumbersome method of giving insulin and do not grant the patient nearly as much freedom in comparison to subcutaneous pump delivery. Whole doses might be neglected in an 'all or none' fashion (viz, the entire shot is foregone but rarely 'restricted) for the reasons described above. By the same token, insulin pumps can prove dangerous because they present a relatively easier administration, rendering patients more susceptible to laxity in terms of dietary schedule liberation and insulin/blood glucose testing.

We can also make the comparison from a chronological diabulimia perspective. Pumps are more likely to be present in an adolescent or adult population (although the proportion of children now treated with pumps is rising). Patients are generally not treated with these devices unless they have demonstrated a certain level of independent competence with insulin calculations and carbohydrate counting – many parents, patients, and even physicians do not feel comfortable with the concept until their child is of substantial age and maturity. As such, pump patients have a dramatically increased autonomy concerning insulin dosing and eating once the transition from insulin injections is made. The role of the parent in diabetes management is gradually if not abruptly curtailed, the shield of external enforcement is eliminated, and the patient becomes more vulnerable to disturbed insulin purging/eating patterns in these more formative stages of their lives.

At the onset of diabulimia, insulin injections and the insulin pump are nigh equivalent in their potential to be neglected. However, due to both the pathophysiology and psychology of the condition, some patients will attempt intermittently to provide themselves insulin or even attempt to regain control of their insulin regimen. Purely theoretically, these efforts (however futile or successful) are perhaps more significantly aided by the pump's resilience, and might even be sabotaged if the patient is only accustomed to using injections. Due to these logistic advantages over the injection system, pump patients who attempt to self-medicate while suffering from diabulimia might encounter fewer impediments or discouragements along the road to recovery. (However, given the potential success of self-medication, diabulimia patients on pumps might appear to be marginally normal. This thereby further confounds the diagnosis and construes the actual prevalence of diabulimia within this population disproportionately lower than the true value.)

Case Descriptions

As indicated above, patterns of insulin omission vary depending on the holistic circumstances inherent to and surrounding the patient. Having outlined the different characteristics of insulin omission and relevant epidemiological statistics, we will present a few brief cases as illustration. These examples are based on real patients, and not necessarily equal in prevalence. (Here, we establish beforehand that the patient suffers from diabulimia/ED-DMT1 – susceptibilities, motivations, and triggers are intentionally excluded for brevity. Diabulimia patients are also rarely as candid as presented here – the didactic is intended to provide information regarding patterns of eating and insulin omission.)

Patient A

A 29-year-old female has an 8 year history of Type I diabetes; she began omitting insulin at the age of 26. At that time, she was on Humalog insulin (short-acting) with an insulin pump, dosing approximately 30 units/day for boluses and 15 units total/day for basal rates. She denied any history of an eating disorder, neither pre- nor post-diagnosis. The course of diabulimia began by omission of approximately 5- to 7-unit boluses for arbitrary snacks and some major meals every few days (usually lunch, but occasionally dinner). This progressed over a few weeks into omitting insulin for every meal except breakfast, but keeping her pump connected such that she received her basal rate each day.

The pattern continued for about 4 months, until she said she felt so physically debilitated that she started to give herself appropriate amounts of insulin again. Her HbA1c was never tested during this time, so there was no quantitative record of the extent of her glucose control. She maintains that her diet and eating habits did not change significantly after the onset of insulin omission, although she did endorse a noticeably elevated appetite.

After three months of proper metabolic control, she began to omit insulin again. In contrast, during this interval she would suspend her pump and eat more than usual for periods of 5-6 days continuously, which she termed "Phase 1." This period was followed by the self-labeled "Phase 2," during which she would reconnect her pump for a few (2-3) days, follow her normal insulin regimen to the letter – but stringently restrict her eating. Phase 1 and Phase 2 were then cycled continuously, the pattern to which she has adhered for approximately the past year. She was admitted thrice to the emergency department for DKA in this interval.

Patient B

A 17-year-old female presents with a history of anorexia nervosa. The eating disorder commenced with restrictive patterns, gradually transitioning to bingeing behaviors (2 times/week) without any compensation after about 7 months. A few months later, she felt some anxiety over gaining weight secondary to the bingeing episodes and began to purge through emesis as well as intense caloric restriction. During this time, she remained gravely underweight, but never received treatment.

This intermittent binge/purge/restriction pattern continued until she was 12 years of age. At this time, she was diagnosed with Type I diabetes after being admitted to the PICU for severe ketoacidosis, where she was treated as inpatient for about a week. After claiming to have gained "about 50 pounds" at the hospital (which further exacerbated her body dysmorphia), she returned home on insulin injections. Her regimen consisted of a Novolog and Levemir combination, which her parents carefully enforced for about 5 months until she was "able to convince them that she could manage by herself." During this period of strict enforcement she returned to severely and consistently restricting her caloric intake/exercising excessively with a few sporadic binge episodes. HbA1c levels ranged between 6-8% during this period.

With her parents no longer monitoring the diabetes regimen, she completely excised the Levemir doses while continuing to restrict her dietary intake. She began to omit insulin for meals in small amounts, about half of each normal dose. Progressively, she eliminated greater ratios of insulin until she was only giving herself about 3-4 units of Novolog directly before she went to sleep. She also used emesis as a purging mechanism, but professed that "it was so much easier to just not take insulin, than the whole rigmarole of throwing up." This behavior consequently faded into disuse, and the above pattern has continued for the past 2 years. At present, the patient administers herself the full amount of insulin for her dinnertime meal, and approximately half the prescribed amount of long-acting, but omits all other injections. She has returned to her binge/purging behavior but the only ICB is insulin omission; she denies restricting her overall caloric intake. Of note, she has gained 8 pounds overall during last three years, though there have been fluctuations within this interval.

Patient C

Patient C is a 21-year-old female diagnosed with Type I diabetes 6 months ago, with no history of a clinical eating disorder. Post-diagnosis she adapted to a new "diabetes diet" but claims to have been incessantly hungry and has experienced multiple instances of nocturnal hypoglycemia. During these excursions, she eats disproportionate amounts (in excess of the quantity necessary to normalize her blood glucose – "almost like a compulsion") and returns to sleep without attempting to check her blood sugar or provide herself requisite insulin. This hypo/hyperglycemic binge episode cycle continued until her apprehension regarding the next potential low blood sugar became so crippling that she has not injected herself at all for the past 2 weeks.

She uses a pen and was not prescribed any long acting insulin. While omitting insulin in these recent weeks, she eats in a self-described "undisciplined" fashion, but rarely has any bingeing episodes. Her HbA1c level at this clinic visit is 10.2%.

Symptoms

The physical symptoms of diabulimia can vary enormously and unpredictably especially given that each person's extent of illness is self-calibrated. There are those generally common to all PWDbs and those appearing on a case-by-case basis. Each also presents along a spectrum of acuity which again must be analyzed according to the individual patient. Also important to consider is the likely presence of other purging behaviors, which might eclipse the observable insulin omission symptoms. In this section, we outline the symptoms experienced by the PWDb and therefore most noticeable to those observing them on a daily (or even clinical) basis. They are essentially passive, made during frequent interpersonal social/familial contact. (Active questioning to flush out the pathology, on the other hand, is covered in Chapter 6: 'Screening,' which is intended primarily for the physician. The following red flags are easier to perceive if the observer spends protracted time with the PWDb.)

Acute

- ***Excessive thirst/urination***

The set of symptoms common to all PWDbs are those experienced by Type I diabetes patients before diagnosis: excessive thirst (polydipsia) accompanied by dry mouth (xerostomia), and excessive urination (polyuria). These are the most acute indications (they can be exhibited within a few hours after induction of hyperglycemia), are constant and continue as long as insulin is foregone, and overlap with the more chronic/specific manifestations described below.[6] The PWDb will appear dehydrated, with

---

[6]   The provenance of diabulimic thirst and urination is quite complex, and includes physiological phenomena such as osmotic diuresis, fluid compartment

dry skin and a peaky pallor. Despite this, they will constantly drink liquids – water, juice – and use the bathroom approximately every 1-3 hours.

Undiagnosed Type I diabetes – a status *physiologically* but not *psychologically* similar to diabulimia – usually presents with the classic "triad" of 1.) polydipsia, 2.) polyuria, and 3.) polyphagia. The former two are feasibly present on the symptomatic spectrum for 'intentional insulin omission executed for weight control,' but a similar statement cannot be issued for the latter. Thirst and urination are largely governed by metabolic processes that the PWDb cannot perturb (unless they intentionally

---

alterations, and elevated levels of anti-diuretic hormone and aldosterone. When sugar builds up in the bloodstream, it creates a hypertonic/hyperosmolar solution that consequently elicits responses from multiple physiological cascades. The first draws water from the intracellular fluid (which by definition has a much lower concentration of glucose), expanding the extracellular volume. Unfortunately, this diluting effort does not restore normal plasma osmolarity, and the serum remains in a hyperosmolar state. The overall increase in serum osmolality 1.) induces a sensation of thirst (diabetic polydipsia and xerostomia) from the hypothalamus, and 2.) shrinks the superoptic magnocellular neurons in the base of the brain, triggering them to release antidiuretic hormone (ADH). ADH acts on the collecting ducts of the kidney to reabsorb water.

Meanwhile, the hyperglycemic plasma is filtered by the kidney glomeruli. If the blood sugar is greater than 160 mg/dl, the sodium-dependent glucose transporters in the proximal convoluted tubules are besieged and allow sugar to spill over into the tubular fluid. As this fluid – now more saturated with glucose solute than to what the nephron is accustomed – passes through the remainder of the tubule, it acts as an osmotic diuretic. The hyperosmolar fluid 'holds' water and prevents a majority of reabsorption by virtue of its concentration, resulting in classic diabetic polyuria.[4] If the PWDb restricts insulin longitudinally, the resulting hyperketonemia functions as a similar diuretic.

As mentioned, the overall rise in plasma osmolarity stimulates release of ADH, which leads to a marginal reclamation of water, but unfortunately is ineffective at restoring plasma volume. Due to perpetually elevated plasma glucose levels, this osmotic diuresis continues, leading to marked dehydration. The body senses this volume depletion and activates the renin-angiotensin-aldosterone cascade - which, like ADH, also proves futile in its efforts to increase sodium and water reabsorption to rectify hypovolemia. The volume depletion also exacerbates ADH release by the paraventricular magnocellular nuclei. In fact, so desperate are these mechanisms in the environment of their impotency that chronic hyperglycemia leads to a state of secondary hyperaldosteronism, concomitant with elevated ADH levels.[2,3]

dehydrate themselves for weight control, which is less than generally viable) and are hence less available for manipulation. On the other hand, polyphagia during the pre-diagnosis state is largely somatic, in that the magnitude of appetite is driven primarily by metabolic and not cognitive requirements/desires/impulses. Unless the patient was already suffering from an eating disorder, then the likelihood is that they were either unattuned to this appetite increase, or aware but not pathologically concerned. Per contra, the presence of disturbed eating in diabulimia renders polyphagia rather useless as a diagnostic symptom because the caloric intake will be psychogenically and not physiologically engineered. The patient will feel hungry due to the body's induced starvation state, but might 1.) intentionally restrict eating despite these signals (and perhaps binge at a later point), or 2.) feel perpetually entitled to eat beyond their caloric necessity given the knowledge that they are not taking insulin.

We must also note that these symptoms are very rapidly reversible, such that a single dose of insulin and adequate effector time will eradicate most conspicuous evidence of thirst or urination. The more chronic symptoms are more difficult to obviate, but simple normalization of the blood sugar – however transient – suppresses the causative physiological dynamics.

- *Gastrointestinal symptoms*

Nausea, vomiting, and abdominal discomfort are frequent presentations of acute hyperglycemia in the setting of ketosis. These symptoms are triggered by hyperosmolar serum glucose concentration and resultant activation of central/peripheral nervous system effectors. However, an equally likely possibility involves mechanical discomfort or overextension of the abdominal wall induced by caloric over-consumption and/or the volume of water that is ingested as a consequence (e.g. in bingeing diabulimia).

Gastrointestinal complaints are not necessarily present in all patients with acute hyperglycemia/ketosis or acute diabulimia – symptoms are physiology-dependent with contributions from both past insulin abuse as well as baseline predisposition. The body's epistat can readjust itself to maintain asymptomatism despite dangerously elevated levels of these compounds.

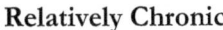

Relatively Chronic

The second set of symptoms is also common to most diabulimia patients and may display characteristics of intermittency, but represents longer-term omission of insulin. The stipulation is that the chronicity as well as severity of the following list of observable symptoms is dependent on the 1.) subtype of diabulimia, as well as 2.) pattern of omission and 3.) duration and extent of insulin restriction. While the materialization, persistence, and grade of these signs might appear random, it is generally true that the greater the abuse, the graver the ramification. (The converse is *not* true – a relatively low level of insulin abuse might still result in consequences of overarching magnitude.) Some patients have testified that the longer they have been omitting insulin, the shorter the interval required to develop symptoms of DKA. (This observation is potentially attributed to progressive, although subclinical, renal deterioration secondary to chronic insulin omission. This results in decreased glomerular filtration rate, impaired expulsion rate of ketones, and hence more rapid accumulation in the bloodstream.) However, all three considerations above must be synthesized in tandem – a bingeing PWDb who has omitted all their insulin for a week might only display a mild case of abdominal pain (or hyperventilation, or cognitive aberration, etc.) as compared to the crippling symptoms of a restricting PWDb who has curtailed small amounts of insulin sporadically for half a decade. Despite these qualifications it is essential that anyone be able to recognize these as potential (but not pathognomonic) indications of diabulimia.

- *Gastroparesis*

This refers to delayed gastric emptying resulting in the stomach pain occurring sporadically with extended periods of hyperglycemia. Nausea and vomiting are also acute presentations of ketotic hyperglycemia, and might be misinterpreted as symptoms of a single episode rather than a reflection of chronic insulin misuse. Gastroparetic indigestion is attributed to damage of the autonomic nerves responsible for stimulating peristalsis, provoked by protracted blood sugar elevation.

This symptom is usually not present on a constant basis for the duration of induced hyperglycemia. Rather, it occurs at dyschronous intervals on a case-by-case basis. Patients are frequently incapacitated during bouts of acute abdominal pain or gastroparetic discomfort, and might present with either diarrhea/constipation and a sensation of premature satiation (with or without nausea and vomiting). Gastroparesis is also a complication that persists even after recovery/normalization of blood sugar, due to the irreparable physical and neurological changes caused by adverse eating/insulin patterns.

- ***Dyspnea***

Respiratory abnormalities are a direct reflection of the metabolic acidosis and ketosis induced by lack of insulin.[7]

Mild hyperventilation is shallow and rapid, and usually signifies less chronic acidosis. It may successfully be obscured and even suppressed, as the drive to expel CO_2 is not quite visceral. It can also be abolished by a short period of basal insulin infusion. The more hazardous respiratory aberration, however, is termed "Kussmaul breathing," a condition that is pathognomic of severe ketoacidosis (blood pH in these cases is usually less than 7.2). This particular ventilation is heavy and deep, and the patient must exert significant effort to take profound breaths while utilizing accessory muscles of breathing (sternocleidomastoids and scalenes). The respiratory rate here is not necessarily elevated, and in fact might be decreased.

---

[7] In this state, glucose is unable to enter the tissues to be used as fuel for glycolysis or oxidative phosphorylation. Consequently, the body must metabolize fat and protein to produce energy. These metabolic processes result in an excessive production of acidic molecules called ketone bodies (which the body normally produces in small amounts collateral to endogenous non-pathological breakdown of dietary and stored fat – but not in the incredible quantity such as present in chronic insulin deficiency). The body's hematological system has established a very efficient buffer system so as to maintain a homeostatic blood pH, using the bicarbonate-carbonic acid molecules:

$$H_2O + CO_2 \leftrightarrow H_2CO_3 \leftrightarrow H^+ + HCO_3$$

An excessive amount of acid (H^+) as produced by the hyper-generation of ketone bodies drives the reaction to the left in order to achieve chemical equilibrium. This results in higher levels of H_2O and CO_2, the latter of which must be eliminated from the body through respiratory exchange in the lungs. The higher pressure of CO_2 in the bloodstream (and therefore alveoli) prompts the hyperventilation witnessed in diabulimia.

Abnormal patterns of breathing are relatively easy to detect, and are also highly indicative of this deadly outcome of chronic hyperglycemia. It is important to be aware of the implications – both mild hyperventilation and conspicuous deep breathing due to DKA are life-threatening, and the patient must be taken to the emergency room as soon as possible. While the PWDb can survive for a relatively longer interval with mild hyperventilation sans therapy, the presence of Kussmaul respirations indicates a highly advanced stage of acidosis rapidly culminating in coma without intervention.

- *Fatigue*

The third chronic symptom is physical/mental exhaustion and corporeal weakness. PWDbs might sleep for abnormally extended periods, and minimal levels of exertion – such as a short walk or climbing a single flight of stairs – might render them breathless and even incapacitated. Energy levels will be subtly or noticeably attenuated; tasks which might previously have been second nature require significant toil, so much so that they are completely foregone. Physical exhaustion can infiltrate cognition, such that the patient's bodily weakness leaves them devoid of energy for mental processes as well. (Distinguish this mental fatigue from the hyperglycemic cognitive anomaly/stupor described later.)

Underlying this symptom is the inability of muscle cells to use glucose for energy. While both endogenous proteins and ketone bodies are available for oxidation, they are vastly inferior to glucose and provide only basal levels of energy on which to subsist. In addition, the PWDb will often experience a cannibalization of muscle mass due to harnessing of myoproteins for alternate metabolic pathways. The loss of lean body mass compounds the detriment to the patient's overall demeanor and vitality. Fatigue is constant and becomes evident after extended periods of time with hyperglycemia.

- *Oral odor*

There is often a mild odor – not precisely halitosis – associated with the breath of a diabetic patient in mild/severe ketoacidosis, described as being "fruity," resembling that of an apple, a pear, or nail polish remover. This is attributed to the presence of high plasma concentrations of circulating acetone, a very volatile type of ketone eliminated primarily through respiration. The urine (or bathroom, after use for urination), also has a similarly sweet/sour odor sometimes mimicking that of alcohol. This sign is hard to perceive, as it is neither obvious, constant, nor readily 'accessible' to the observer. Experienced physicians, however, can recognize the smell as soon as they enter the room.

- *Cognitive anomaly*

This is one of the most subtle dispositions, and can present either acutely or chronically. Hyperglycemia has been shown to reduce both acute attention span and mental capacity, while promoting dysphoria and anxiety.[18] Patients might slur speech, verbalize non-linear thought processes, demonstrate no insight into their condition, and be unable to effectively engage in conversation. Some patients have described this effect as a sensation of "mental fogginess," "incapability of focusing on any specific subject," "bizarre loss of immediate factoids," "blurry inability to remember things, which mysteriously can be recalled after the necessity for recollection has passed." Proustian (involuntary) recollection is largely preserved, but the patient can display conspicuous problems with voluntary memory. (A useful confirmation in underage patients is a reduced scholastic performance.) In some instances cognitive abilities are so markedly impaired that the patient is qualitatively dysfunctional – so devoid of acuity that they walk around in a "dazed and glazed" fashion. This altered state of consciousness can even approach stupor and delirium (in which case the threshold for suspicion of DKA must be extremely low). Unfortunately, mental aberration does not completely resolve post-recovery – patients testify that memory loss and certain cognitive impairments persist for years.

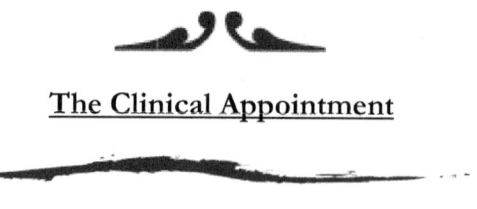

The Clinical Appointment

Interview

The past medical histories of insulin-omitting eating disordered patients (and in some cases, non-insulin-omitting eating-disordered diabetics) frequently show multiple hospitalizations for diabetic ketoacidosis (DKA). A quick glance at the actual dates for past clinic visits (especially those to endocrinology) will reveal erratic and extended intervals between appointments, excessive cancellations, and no-shows. Patients with eating disorders are generally ambivalent towards the clinical environment, which 1.) engenders fear of repercussion, and 2.) is a potential nidus towards relinquishing command to agents who might reverse their attempts at weight/diet control. Quantitative measurements reflecting compliance which are garnered during the appointment, such as weight or HbA1c levels, contribute to this pattern. Evading clinical presence is not specific to the autonomous population – younger patients also endeavor to escape physician contact, most often through parental manipulation.

The patient's history, particularly the most recent, might show irregular menstruation or frank amenorrhea: an indication that the body cannot shoulder the burden of a fetus given the present nutritional and physiological status. Termed 'hypogonadotropic hypogonadism' or 'hypothalamic-pituitary amenorrhea,' the pituitary gland fails to secrete the hormones necessary to signal the ovaries (or testes) to in turn secrete the secondary hormones for ovulation, conception, and uterine preparation for pregnancy. Pre-pubertal and pubertal age patients likewise exhibit signs of delayed sexual and growth maturation – inadequate nutritional status and hormonal derailment (especially decreased growth hormone levels) are complications of chronic hyperglycemia. Bone and weight growth curves will manifest a 'falling off the curve' i.e. a crossing to lower percentiles (largely in the restrictive diabulimia subpopulation).

A review of systems might reveal the following (granted the patient is honest with the clinician):

➢ hair loss (lack of nutrients from caloric deficiency)
➢ swollen face/extremities (edema due to alternating cycles of insulin omission and compliance, or progressive kidney dysfunction with low blood protein levels)
➢ blurry vision (cycles of hyperglycemia/euglycemia lead to hemodynamic derangement in the fundus humors)
➢ dental caries, acute/chronic periodontitis, degeneration/bleeding/inflammation of the teeth and gingiva (sequelae of chronic acidosis, hyperglycemia and subsequent

bacterial colonization, vitamin deficiencies from macronutritional restriction)

➤ delayed healing of bruises and/or increased bruising (poor vascular supply secondary to hyperglycemia, impaired immune function)

➤ delayed onset or abrupt cessation/irregularity of menses

➤ prominent vasculature, especially cervical veins

➤ recurrent infections due to 1.) bacteria – metabolic aberration results in weakened immune defenses (otitis media, urinary tract/pyelonephritis – autonomic neuropathy leads to incomplete bladder emptying, overflow incontinence with elevated post-void residual urine causing infection), or 2.) fungi – most frequently *Candida albicans*, which can be oral/systemic (search for cracking at the corners of the lips – 'cheilitis') – and recurrent vaginal yeast infections. These organisms are opportunistic – uncontrolled diabetes is a state of immunocompromise, and glycemic derangement favors their pathological proliferation despite commensal existence in the mucosal flora. The hyperalimentation of binge-purge diabulimia also contributes.) *Mucor/Rhizopus* species infections (oral and rhinocerebral abcesses) are also recognized (although rare) sequelae of uncontrolled diabetes – these are far more invasive and require hospitalization.

➤ pathological bone fractures or breaks with minimal trauma (decreased bone density/osteopenia/osteoporosis secondary to 1.) chronic malnutrition with calcium and vitamin D malabsorption, 2.) metabolic acidosis – excess H+ is buffered by bone breakdown, 3.) hypoestrogenic state induced by eating disorders)

➤ dizziness and postural hypotension (acute and chronic autonomic nervous system dysfunction, as well as perpetuated dehydration)

➤ cramps, shaking, or spasms/fasciculations due to electrolyte abnormalities induced by hyperglycemic diuresis and loss in the urine/gastrointestinal tract

➤ numbness in the fingers or toes (destruction of sensory nerves in the extremities)

➤ parched/flaking skin (chronic dehydration)

➤ delayed reaction time ('hyperglycemic faze')

The belief that individuals with ED-DMT1/diabulimia are underweight is an unfortunate misconception engendered by observations of the general eating-disordered population, and vernacular media-perpetuated definitions of "anorexia" and "bulimia."

A related myth propagated through the Type I community is that diabulimia necessarily entails substantial weight loss (as presents prior to diagnosis of Type I). Many people with a rudimentary Type I repertoire believe that if a diabetic patient is not receiving insulin – intentionally or unintentionally – they will accordingly lose dramatic body mass. Consistent with such rationale, if their weight is reasonably static then their insulin dosing must be sufficient, yes? No. There is an outstanding psychological difference between the pre-diagnosis period (when the patient is not aware of their insulin deficiency, let alone its use as a viable purging tool) and the period of diabulimia (where the patient manipulates insulin doses prior to or subsequent to adverse psychosomatic eating). There is little to no psychogenic contribution towards the caloric intake of pre-diagnosis *diabetes* patients – while they eat in quantities far above standard requirements due to their insulin-deficient starvation state, they generally cease when satiation is attained. The caloric intake of *diabulimia* patients, on the other hand, is dictated by conscious and unconscious mental processes. A binge, for example, is the multifactorial outcome of adverse physiological dynamics and underlying psychosomatic mandates – none of which are appreciably present in a pre-diagnosed non-eating-disordered patient. As such, Type I diabetic patients with eating disorders actually have normal to high BMI's (due to intermittent periods of proper insulin/glycemic control which have not been compensated for by concomitant caloric normalization, cyclical edema, and the tropic effect of insulin). Diabulimia renders them more prone to long-term overall weight *gain*. The myth of "diabulimia patients being skinny" or "shedding pounds quickly," is actually quite dangerous, as it could erroneously eliminate diabulimia from the differential diagnosis. It is a potent psychological confound on the part of the clinician, and must emphatically be underscored.

(The above qualification applies largely to bingeing PWDbs, as restrictive patients are not likely to overeat to a salient extent. Restrictive patients constitute a minority of individuals with diabulimia, which has yet regrettably done little to debunk the reigning fallacy of diabulimic weight loss.)

Physical Exam

There are certain bedside signs with which the physician should be familiar in order to even include diabulimia in the differential diagnosis. One of the most important clinical parameters is a patient's external appearance, demeanor, and affect. This element and its implications are frequently far more enlightening than those offered by the stethoscope and lab results combined. Eating-disordered diabetic patients (especially the diabulimia subset) tend to appear lethargic and dejected, with overall flat affect. Their cognitive function is depressed, their movements inhibited, their pallor anemic, peaky, and perhaps even jaundiced.

An abbreviated mental status exam can help to elucidate the cognitive anomalies concomitant with either acute or chronic high blood sugar. Questions pertaining to orientation, time, place, and situation (such as "Where are we?" "Why are we here?" "What year is it?" or "When were you born?") should be assessed for coherence and aptness of response, and any deviations appropriately noted. Patients might be either expressly unable to answer, respond with inaccuracies, or have acute difficulty in addressing the inquiries. Articulation is occasionally impaired, rendering somewhat slurred phonemes, and generally compromised acuity. The patient might inadvertently mistake some minor details, such as recollection of numbers (for example, an insulin dose provided during the appointment), or incorrect repetition of letters, dates, etc. No matter how trivial, this type of subtlety should also be duly noted. Often these seemingly inconsequential observations are the only intimations that there something awry.

The actual physical exam might demonstrate chronic or acute sequelae of metabolic derangements and electrolyte/fluid abnormalities. Vital signs reveal low blood pressure and/or orthostasis; thready, rapid, or irregular pulses; temperature trends towards the lower end of normal. Skin and mucous membranes are dry, conjunctiva 'muddy' and injected. Tooth enamel is eroded, gingiva and salivary glands swollen. The abdomen might be tender to palpation in a nonspecific pattern secondary to gastroparesis. Examination of the extremities demonstrates hypotonia, hyporeflexia, muscle spasm, and areas of slight to gross pitting edema. If the PWDb is 'advanced,' peripheral neuropathy in the 'stocking' distribution (as manifest by impaired vibration sensation and/or abnormal microfilament testing) and pathologies in the optic fundus might be perceived.

The above physical symptoms are not diabulimia-specific, and when manifest are most likely auxiliary to other non-insulin-omitting purging characteristics. As compensatory behaviors frequently 'travel in packs' their presence can alert the onlooker to insulin omission. As such, clinicians should also familiarize themselves with the indications of vomiting/laxative/diuretic abuse – incorporating any piece into the puzzle functions a long way in unearthing a patient suffering from diabulimia. For example, patients who vomit as an ICB will typically use the bathroom soon after completing a meal, have discolored and damaged teeth from upended gastric acids, and knuckle calluses from manual induction of the gag reflex (Russell's sign). We will not enumerate them all here.

Noting any of these symptoms (or lack thereof) and analyzing them in isolation is dangerous, leading to a slew of both false positives and negatives. All observations must be synthesized within the patient's larger context to enhance their predictive value – demographic likelihood, presence/absence of suspicious insulin use, symptoms of acute/chronic hyperglycemia, demeanor, and such. Much of what we have described is highly *sensitive* for diabulimia, but not *specific*; it is therefore essential that observers refrain from leaping to premature conclusions.

Laboratory Values

Laboratory diagnostic tools can also be helpful in the process of narrowing the differential diagnosis to diabulimia, as well as commencing treatment of any complications that might already be present. However, without knowledge of the overt symptoms described above, the patient might never even 1.) make it to the clinic for evaluation, 2.) impress upon the doctor (intentionally or unintentionally) that they are suffering from a diabulimia-related condition. Similar to the symptoms/signs described in previous sections of this chapter, laboratory values are highly sensitive but absolutely not specific; they are presented for 'gestalt' purposes.

HbA1c

The short-term diagnostic workup for a patient suspected of diabulimia should include at the very least the glycosylated hemoglobin, which will most likely be elevated past the standard 6.5% therapeutic goal – the degree of deviation varies depending upon each patient's specific eating patterns. Restrictive PWDbs are startlingly capable of remaining peripheral to this delineation. (In general, many exceptions trending towards clinical normality are characteristic of this subgroup; the decreased caloric intake imposes a ceiling for attainable hyperglycemia which is actually conducive to glucose homeostasis – although toxic for other systems). The same is much more difficult for a bingeing PWDb – the A1c might be on the higher end of normal to undetectably elevated (i.e. usually >14%, when the POCT machine cannot even register the amount of glycosylated hemoglobin as the levels are so far removed from their range of statistical sensitivity). Baseline and historical hemoglobin levels must also be accounted for: a patient who has regularly maintained an A1c of 8.5% might not feasibly be suspected of diabulimia, but a patient who presents with an A1c of 8.5% after a past history of 6.5% must elicit concern (unless, of course, there are extenuating circumstances such as concurrent stress or illness).

A common fallacy is that elevated HbA1c levels are diagnostic of intentional insulin omission if an eating disorder is present, and conversely that elevated HbA1c levels are a prerequisite for diagnosis of diabulimia. Patients with eating disorders, especially those falling into the bulimia or bingeing subcategories, are rendered powerfully susceptible to producing hyperglycemia sans intentional insulin restriction. Uncontrolled eating, as occurs during a binge, almost by default relinquishes any calculation for insulin doses. Even if the patient attempts to bolus themselves, they will use gross approximations of carbohydrate intake and risk significant departures from normoglycemia – both above and below the acceptable range. The patient who vomits or uses another purging method will have no perception of the actual amount of metabolized carbohydrates due to the imprecise expulsion of caloric intake. As such, bingeing is not even necessary for this miscalculation to occur – a patient who purges through vomiting after a normal or reduced caloric intake (viz, a "restrictive" eating disordered diabetic patient) would experience similar repercussions. The prospectively resultant hypoglycemia can lead to 1.) medical emergency, and 2.) perpetuated fear of low blood sugar inspiring insulin omission during future binge episodes. On the other hand, the potential hyperglycemia – induced post-binge, binge/purge, or just purge – can effect drastic changes in glycosylated hemoglobin if they occur frequently enough (as well as a potent "trigger" for attempting to use insulin to negate the excessive binge intake). Thus, an eating-disordered patient might have incredibly high HbA1c levels despite express absence of *intentional* insulin omission.

Likewise, PWDbs are quite capable of sustaining reasonable HbA1c measurements – this is due in part to the biokinetic mechanisms of hemoglobin glycosylation, and also the particular pattern of insulin omission to which the patient subscribes. If they skip an insulin shot once a week, or go for an entire day without insulin sporadically but relatively infrequently, the transgression will not register in the HbA1c. Such an issue again raises the question of clinical criteria – after which delineation does "skipping an insulin dose for one meal" become a clinical problem? Further complicating matters is the fact that both endocrinology and psychiatry teams will have different measurements specifying the presence or absence of pathology.

None of this is to imply that elevated HbA1c levels should be overlooked within the overarching mental health context. Sometimes it is the last jigsaw in the puzzle of distinguishing diabulimia, especially given the appropriate demographic and clinical observations. We provide these important qualifications in order that no subset be overlooked or misunderstood.

Glucose

Serum glucose will be elevated – some patients can even reach blood levels above 1000mg/dl (serum). On the other hand, a normal level is also feasible (although much less likely) if the PWDb had temporarily dosed themselves with short-acting insulin before sample collection to evade detection. Depending on the chronicity of the duplicitous 'dosing,' the urine glucose might also be normalized.

Ketones

Urine ketones will also be elevated – often markedly greater than 100 mg/dl. Although patients precariously navigate the edge of ketoacidotic emergency, they can survive for a period of time with ketonemia and ketonuria without symptoms; the only way to confirm their presence in such circumstances is through diagnostic testing. Ketone measurements are generally less vulnerable to endogenous manipulation with 'preparatory correctional' insulin dosing. Physiological elimination of ketones, if not performed in an inpatient unit with intravenous fluids, is generally a chronic renal/respiratory process that can take days to rectify even under restored orthoglycemia/orthoinsulinemia. A short time with insulin will normalize the blood glucose but cannot immediately circulating ketones. Falsifying a urine sample is possible; patients most commonly dilute it with water, which makes the concentration of ketones and glucose appear less than the true amount. For this reason, a urine specific gravity is sometimes concomitantly checked with the sample to screen for manipulation. The specific gravity is also highly useful to trend during outpatient or inpatient eating disorder/diabulimia treatment, as it can elucidate 1.) attempts at 'water-loading' to hoodwink the physician into believing that they have manifested appropriate weight gain between clinic intervals (in which the specific gravity will be low, indicating lack of urine-concentrating processes), or 2.) whether dehydration is contributing to apparent weight loss (in which the specific gravity will be high, indicating urine concentration. This might signify dehydration as a possible etiology of decreased measured weight in the clinic, rather than a loss of true body mass).

Lipid Panel

The physician will not (and should not) order full laboratory panels executed on whole blood/serum for the express purpose of confirming a diabulimia-related condition, unless merited for other reasons during the standard Type I diabetes "check-in" appointment. They are not likely to elucidate much, as it is difficult to 'catch' diabulimia within one discrete lab window; however, there are some clues that can be garnered from these tests. The fasting lipid panel might demonstrate abnormally elevated total/serum triglycerides, LDL, and VLDL cholesterols. Chronic insulin deficiency relieves the inhibition on adipocytic lipolysis, leading to impaired hepatic clearance and higher circulating triglycerides. Dietary patterns of insulin-omitting patients, especially bingeing PWDbs, are also likely to consist of macronutrient ratios favoring those elements detrimental to lipid levels, such as saturated and/or trans fats. The negative predictive value of this observation in regards to diabulimia is more distinct if the patient is younger, ie in an age group where high cholesterol/triglycerides are not usually apparent.

Electrolytes

The electrolyte panel (usually performed in the inpatient setting, perhaps for DKA or another presenting pathology) will also show some particular abnormalities. Serum potassium levels might be borderline to increased, despite decreased total body stores of the mineral. Insulin in normal titers shuttles this mineral intracellularly, and in the insulin-deficient state leads to increased blood levels. Patients can also become hyponatremic with significant degrees of hyperglycemia. Acute kidney injury due to critical dehydration leads to higher-than-baseline levels of BUN and creatinine, especially in DKA. If the patient has omitted insulin for an appreciable amount of time (which can range from 12 hours to a few days, depending on the particular patient or the magnitude of omission), their serum pH will be decreased and the anion gap increased due to a predominance of acidic ketone bodies in circulation. Likewise, bicarbonate will also be decreased (although depending on chronicity, might be normal due to renal compensation for the metabolic acidosis). Bicarbonate levels are likely to be low if the patient uses emesis as an inappropriate compensatory behavior due to loss of gastric acids. Secondary to dehydration and resultant hemoconcentration, the hematocrit level might also be elevated.

References:

1.) Katz, Murray A. "Hyperglycemia-Induced Hyponatremia — Calculation of Expected Serum Sodium Depression." New England Journal of Medicine 289.16 (1973): 843-44.

2.) Zerbe, R. L., F. Vinicor, and G. L. Robertson. "Plasma Vasopressin in Uncontrolled Diabetes Mellitus." Diabetes 28.5 (1979): 503-08.

3.) Nestler, J. E., C. O. Barlascini, G. A. Tetrault, M. J. Fratkin, J. N. Clore, and W. G. Blackard. "Increased Transcapillary Escape Rate of Albumin in Nondiabetic Men in Response to Hyperinsulinemia." Diabetes 39.10 (1990): 1212-217.

4.) Gennari, F.John, and Jerome P. Kassirer. "Osmotic Diuresis." New England Journal of Medicine 291.14 (1974): 714-20.

5.) Takii M, Uchigata Y, Nozaki T, Nishikata H, Kawal K, Komaki G, Iwamoto Y, Kubok C. Classification of Type 1 Diabetic Females With Bulimia Nervosa Into Subgroups According to Purging Behavior. Diabetes Care 2001; 25: 1571-575.

6.) Goebel-Fabbri A, Fikkan J, Franko D, Pearson K, Anderson B, Weinger K. Insulin Restriction and Associated Morbidity and Mortality in Women with Type 1 Diabetes. Diabetes Care 2008 Mar;31(3):415-9

7.) Polonsky W, Anderson B, Lohrer P, Aponte J, Jacobson A, Cole C. Insulin Omission in women with IDDM. Diabetes Care 1994: 1178-185.

8.) Rydall A, Rodin G, Olmsted M, Devenyi R, Daneman D. Disordered Eating Behavior and Microvascular Complications in Young Women with Insulin-Dependent Diabetes Mellitus. New England Journal of Medicine 1997; 336: 1849-854.

9.) Daneman, D. Eating Disorders in Adolescent Girls and Young Women with Type I Diabetes. Diabetes Spectrum 2002; 15 : 83-105.

10.) Goebel-Fabbri A, Fikkan J, Franko D, Pearson K, Anderson B, Weinger K. Insulin Restriction and Associated Morbidity and Mortality in Women with Type 1 Diabetes. Diabetes Care (2007).

11.) The Diabetes Control and Complications Trial Research Group. The effect of intensive treatment of diabetes on the development and progression of long-term complications in insulin-dependent diabetes mellitus. New England Journal of Medicine 1993: 329:977-86.

12.) Peveler R, Fairburn C, Boller I, Dunger D. Eating Disorders in Adolescents with IDDM. A controlled study. Diabetes Care 1992; 1356-360.

13.) Daneman D, Olmsted M, Rydall A, Maharaj S, Rodin G. Eating Disorders in Young Women with Type 1 Diabetes: Prevalence, Problems and Prevention. Hormone Research 1998; 50: 79-86.

14.) Bryden, K, Niel A, Mayou R, Peveler R, Fairburn C, Dunger D. Eating Habits, Body Weight, and Insulin Misuse. Diabetes Care 1999; 22 : 1956-960.

15.) Fairburn, C, Peveler R, Davies B, Mann JI, Mayou R. Eating Disorders in Young Adults with Insulin Dependent Diabetes Mellitus: A Controlled Study. British Medical Journal 1991; 303.

16.) Hsu, Y., B. Chen, M. Huang, S. Lin, M. Lin. Disturbed Eating behaviors in Taiwanese Adolescents with Type I Diabetes Mellitus: a comparative study. Pediatric Diabetes 2008: 1-8.

17.) Biggs M, Basco M, Patterson G, Raskin P. Insulin Witholding for weight control in women with diabetes. Diabetes Care 1994; 1186-189.

18.) Ferguson, S. C., A. Blane, P. Perros, R. J. McCrimmon, J. J.K. Best, J. Wardlaw, I. J. Deary, and B. M. Frier. "Cognitive Ability and Brain Structure in Type 1 Diabetes: Relation to Microangiopathy and Preceding Severe Hypoglycemia." Diabetes 52.1 (2003): 149-56.

19.) Laffel, L. Ketone bodies: a review of physiology, pathophysiology and application of monitoring to diabetes Diabetes Metabolism Reviews Rev 1999; 15: 412-426

20.) Mosley, Philip E. "Bigorexia: Bodybuilding and Muscle Dysmorphia." European Eating Disorders Review 17.3 (2009): 191-98.

21.) Rome, E. S., S. Ammerman, D. S. Rosen, R. J. Keller, J. Lock, K. A. Mammel, J. O'Toole, J. M. Rees, M. J. Sanders, S. M. Sawyer, M. Schneider, E. Sigel, and T. J. Silber. "Children and Adolescents With Eating Disorders: The State of the Art." Pediatrics 111.1 (2003): E98-108. Print.

22.) Svensson, M., I. Engström, and J. Åman. "Higher Drive for Thinness in Adolescent Males with Insulin-dependent Diabetes Mellitus Compared with Healthy Controls." Acta Paediatrica 92.1 (2003): 114-17. Print.

23.) Rosen, David, and Committee on Adolescence. "Identification and Management of Eating Disorders in Children and Adolescents." Pediatrics 126 (2010): 1240-1253

CHAPTER 5

EXECUTION

Diabulimia and social life are not mutually exclusive. But they are difficult to juggle simultaneously, if you want to keep the condition expressly hidden. People are by default not admirably observant, but there are some things that we cannot easily conceal even from the most cataracted of eyes.

I drove around in the city with my friends once, visiting different landmarks — Chinatown, the zoo, a restaurant for lunch. I tried to be smooth about my bathroom visits — once saying I needed to wash the sticky residue from my hands after a meal, later following a friend after she mentioned she needed to use the toilet. Everyone was annoyed when I asked if we could stop by a gas station or a Starbucks before entering the freeway for the long drive home. "You have such a thimble-sized bladder," someone grumbled in irritation. Then there was the thirst, easy enough to deflect if your Camelback was voluminous enough. But refilling was always a problem — free water unfortunately does not exist every three city blocks unless you're willing to pay for a Subway sandwich that you don't want anyway.

Those stipulations were easy enough, relatively if that. But what do you tell people when you can't walk more than 2 blocks, climb three steps, lift a bag of picnic groceries without feeling breathless? Without feeling palpitations, without a dreadful sensation of exhaustion, your eyes bloodshot and face drawn in profoundly acute stress? What do you do when a quiet stroll down the banks of a lake leaves you so utterly spent that you fall asleep in the car while everyone else enjoys a rousing conversation on the politics of seafood sustainability?

I have tried. I have tried defeating all of these, to meld myself into fibers of normality that the social tapestry has dictated. I think such efforts are to some avail, and those who are clever enough can pass by with their pathologies unnoticed. But I think this is precisely why I relate this to you — that I did it so well, that I was too smart for my own good, that I obliterated any chance of ever getting help by virtue of this criminally-worthy deception. Because nobody really knew, and by the same token nobody understood how truly serious my problem was...

Towards Recognition

<u>NOTE</u>: Please do not proceed if you are a currently 1.) an active diabulimia patient, 2.) in an unstable psychological condition, 3.) in a period of fresh recovery, 4.) are in any manner uncomfortable with your status. This chapter contains potentially triggering information.

P eople with particular illnesses sometimes attempt to conceal both the reason for and the existence of that sickness. For example, some patients with eczema or psoriasis will wear garments with long sleeves and pants so as not to reveal their afflictions; people suffering from depression might erect facades of mannerism or tone in order to appear completely ordinary in mood. Patients with diabulimia more often than not will try to do the same, using deception and manipulation to project an image of normality.

In no way is this chapter or the next ("Screening") designed to portray the PWDb as a common criminal under investigation, or a refractory child in need of disciplinary action. Diabulimia is far more complex than these superficial deceptions and subterfuges, and patients cannot be treated as if they are no better than a garden-variety pickpocket. However, we cannot deny that these do exist, and the ability to recognize them is a sensitive (although not specific) tool towards detection.

The degree of masquerading varies. Some patients are highly obsessive and intently focused on posing as normal, adherent diabetic patients. Some might hide their practices reasonably well but allow a few oversights to pass unfiltered (by virtue that this endeavor is not at the forefront of consciousness). Still others will not care enough to even concern themselves with cheating; these patients either 1.) do not find concealment expressly necessary, 2.) are exhausted and 'burnt out,' or 3.) have come to terms with their family/environment/physician discovering or already knowing.

The reasons underlying duplicity are not always as straightforward as they appear. Of course, the primary motivation is to cultivate a façade of compliance in order to satisfy a proximal environment, but, as with other eating disorders, there is also an element of deep shame. The sensations of guilt, inadequacy, low self-esteem, remorse – if present, are profound, and the PWDb will go to great lengths to conceal these perceived transgressions.

Type I diabetes is a very intercalative condition, and if the PWDb wants to successfully obscure any insulin-omitting practices, they must look to blood sugar testing, insulin administration, eating habits, urination frequency, and HbA1c testing. There is a daily need to hide diabulimia from the immediate family or living environment, an intermittent (if slightly less incumbent) prompting to hide it from the social group, and an absolute long-term requirement to conceal it from the endocrinologist.

Short-term Deception

In the short-term, the patient with diabulimia needs to camouflage the nuances in which their lifestyle diverges from those of an otherwise conventional diabetic patient. This is to convince people central to daily living: parents, spouses, partners, siblings, children. These are most often familiar with the patient's regimen of blood sugar testing and insulin dosing, and would thus notice any aberrations in practice.

Blood Glucose Monitoring

The first arena is that of the blood sugar monitor. In recent years the advent of the Continuous Glucose Monitoring (CGM) system has made the traditional blood sugar testing kit appear obsolete, but it remains an integral constituent of even the relatively small proportion of patients using this technology. Of note, these new modalities are significantly more difficult to thwart due to their autonomous nature (viz., one-time subcutaneous insertion) and continuous readout. It is consequently more difficult to fabricate blood sugar values with the CGM compared to the conventional glucometer. Secondary to these features, PWDbs (especially those over 18 years) will generally opt out of using it for the purposes of camouflage. Past history might include initial use of the CGM during a period of presumably normal psychology, followed by severance (the date of which is a supposed indicator of gradual diabulimia onset). However, this is not necessarily true in patients attempting to self-medicate during efforts towards recovery, who often vacillate between periods of acceptable metabolic control and insulin omission. Although clinical studies to date have only demonstrated a benefit of the CGM in adult populations over 25 years, some adolescents/children might have been placed on the technology earlier and still currently use it in their diabetes management secondary to maintenance of clinical continuity or parental mandate.[7] Patients who develop diabulimia in these circumstances also find it necessary to execute techniques of subterfuge. Thus, both subpopulations of patients might demonstrate particularities and intimations of insulin misuse in CGM readouts.

The following discussion pertains to monitoring in a setting *without* the CGM, but details of duplicity with this method of glucose testing will be discussed later in the chapter. Obviously, a complete lack of or a dramatic reduction in blood glucose testing is indicative of insulin omission, and should elicit concern. Holding a basic operational knowledge of a conventional glucose testing kit is essential, as these are the principal features manipulated by the patient. The test strip is pretreated (by the manufacturer) with a chemical solution containing a glucose oxidase or glucose dehydrogenase enzyme. The patient inserts this strip into the main apparatus of the kit, and proceeds to apply a 2-3 millimeter diameter drop of fresh capillary blood from a finger pad or a forearm to the edge of the strip. A precise volume of blood is drawn into the strip via capillary action, and the quantity of glucose in the sample reacts with the enzyme on the strip.[8]

As such, there are a few ways by which this circuit is subverted. First, liquids other than blood can be inserted into the test strip in order to

---

8   Glucose itself in solution is not an electrolyte (it is not broken down into charged ions), necessitating the presence of glucose oxidase on the strip. As its name implies, this enzyme catalyzes the oxidation of glucose into hydrogen peroxide and D-glucono-δ-lactone, the process of which requires a flow of electrons to be harnessed for quantification. Depending on the glucose monitor manufacturer, various components of this reaction are measured and transposed in different fashions. The end result is an electronic display of the blood glucose concentration in mg/dl (US) or mmol/L (Europe). The main apparatus is calibrated (by both the manufacturer and at certain intervals by the patients themselves) to reflect accurate glucose concentrations.

obtain a viable 'blood sugar' reading. The most intuitive approach, and perhaps the most common, is a mixture of pre-cleansing liquid (either water or ethanol) – and blood. Patients will feign to wash their hands prior to testing; alternatively they will excoriate a few fingers with an alcohol swab. They will then prematurely extract a drop of blood and allow it to mix with the vestiges of intentionally retained water or alcohol. The endogenous blood is effectively diluted, fabricating a blood sugar lower than the actual value. (Although logical, plain water will not function for this purpose, as it prompts an "Error" or "LO" (monitor-speak for 'low') reading, indicating that the amount of glucose was completely undetectable. The same principle applies to pure alcohol.)

The glucometer's calibration liquid, a synthetic solution provided by the particular glucose kit manufacturer, is another exploited substance. It is meant to be used at specific intervals to ensure that the machine is providing readouts in the proper input-output range. The PWDb may simply replace their own blood with this substance and continue to pretend that their glucose levels are totally normal. A family member should note that a distinctive feature of this byzantine approach is the presence of readings that are often repetitive and very narrow in range. Take, for example, the following set of glucose levels at 9am, 12pm, 4pm, 8pm, and 11pm, respectively: 113, 117, 109, 113, 109, 109, 120. This is only meant as qualitative illustration, and can obviously be manipulated further by the patient – i.e. by diluting the sample or adding materials (see below) in order to widen the range of readings and further perpetuate the appearance of a realistic spectrum. Onlookers must also be leery if the diabetic requests new blood glucose kits more often than seems necessary (these are now very readily available – oftentimes free with a prescription – and pose a dramatically reduced financial investment as compared to previous years). The purpose of this is usually to harvest the calibration solutions provided with each new kit, which are actually adequate for 1-2 years unless they are being harnessed inappropriately.

Another way in which patients sabotage the glucose kit is by using the most readily available alternative liquid saliva. Saliva, if not for any reason other than that it is the receptacle for orally ingested glucose and other molecules, sometimes provides a suitable glucose value. This is actually a very commonly utilized medium, as it generates a very wide range of falsified blood glucose values (not to mention the convenience of its accessibility). If the PWDb coats the surface of the mouth with glucose molecules – for example, by eating or drinking virtually anything containing a simple sugar, such as fruit juice, milk, or a slice of bread, the glucose concentration of the saliva is altered, and thus, the reading registered by the central apparatus. A logbook of values taken from a kit doctored in this style is alarmingly realistic and almost statistically randomized – the practiced PWDb can sharpen these levels even further based on their particular degree of charade.

There are obviously myriad other solutions and schemes used to falsify blood sugar readings. Patients will dilute sugary drinks and use nail polish to mimic the hue of blood.[4] One method of doctoring glucose values that does not involve spurious liquids is waiting until the blood sugar is within range, and then testing it multiple times so as to construct a 'history.' The resulting pattern is neither statistically nor chronologically realistic, but for the inexperienced eye appears to be completely acceptable due to the normal readings.

Lack of finger markings is also a stigmata of diabulimia. Patients with diabetes usually develop clusters of dark pinprick dots from lancet penetration on the pads or peripheries of their fingers. These markings usually take 1-2 months to disappear, and an outstanding absence indicates a gross lack of bona fide glucose testing – the patient is either generating counterfeit readings or not bothering to deal with glucose testing at all.

If diabulimia is suspected, watching the [underage] patient closely as they execute every step of the blood sugar testing sequence is crucially important. They will do their utmost to stall and distract; unfortunately, a sideward glance is literally the interval of time required to institute their chosen technique for falsification.

Insulin Administration

The second area to veil is the insulin regimen. The same stipulation applies here: there is marked heterogeneity based on 1.) the conscientiousness of the PWDb, 2.) particular pattern of insulin omission and eating habits, and 3.) insulin administration modality.

The highly meticulous PWDb might effect various simulations so to stifle any concerns regarding their compliance level. Such pretenses mainly involve a "going through the motions" of diabetes without genuinely executing them. This is rare, however, and most patients fall into laxity as either an acute result of the metabolic and mental derangements of diabulimia, or develop an attitude of disinterest towards fraudulence as the illness adopts a chokehold. If the patient becomes sloppy in their agenda of disguise, there will be a few signs which should raise red flags.

The particular pattern of insulin omission is also a key factor in the way a PWDb conceals their pathology. For example, if a patient on the pump completely omits the insulin required for breakfast and lunch but still receives their basal insulin rate and the dosage for dinner, they might still feel it necessary to keep their pump connected for the majority of the day. By the same token, a patient on insulin injections who deliberately underdoses themselves for each meal (e.g. 15 units instead of the requisite 30) would stand in stark contrast to someone on a similar dosing schedule who omits the entirety of their dose. The former would still appear to give themselves insulin, whereas the latter will manifest little to no injection 'activity.'

- *Injections/Pens*

The most common modalities of insulin administration at present are injections/pens, and the pump. Insulin injections are relatively easy to forego, and technical deceit is rarely necessary. Akin to the express observation of blood sugar testing, doubt in the veracity of management might be aroused if there is a complete deficiency or decrease in activity surrounding needles, alcohol swabs, or insulin vials. However, a more conscientious PWDb often pre-empts this skepticism by creating a charade of injecting themselves. They might refuse to take shots in public, insisting on injecting in privacy while feigning anxiety or embarrassment. Some stonewalling is also incorporated so as to divert or exhaust the observer into losing concentration: pretending to find the perfect spot for injection, extensive time to sanitize the skin, saying they are unable to withdraw the correct amount of insulin, cannot eliminate bubbles from the vial/pen, feigning fear of piercing the flesh, and the like. As soon as all attention in their direction is eliminated, the insulin is squirted out of the needle or pen in the blink of an eye – into air, cloth, onto the floor. Some insulins, especially the short-acting lispro formulation, have a distinctive volatile odor which might be perceptible if suddenly exposed (i.e. relieved from standard encapsulation in a vial, syringe, pen, or subcutaneous tissue) in this fashion.

- ***Pump***

The pump is a horse of a different color. The administration of insulin using this technology is far subtler and often consists only of pressing a few buttons on the beeper-sized apparatus connected subcutaneously to the patient. One of the original premises of the device was enhancing logistic management – e.g., increasing convenience for the patient, minimizing the recalcitrance of transporting the equipment associated with insulin injections, and generally tapering the invasive nature of diabetes therapy (among myriad other important medical features). In the case of diabulimia, these beneficial features might actually prove counterproductive as they not only 1.) by default drastically diminish the observer's awareness of the device and consequently any aberrations in usage, but also 2.) promote insulin omission by virtue of the relative ease of insulin management. Although the pump as insulin therapy can exist much less conspicuously than injections, diligent surveillance might yet elucidate a few peculiar features.

First of all, the patient is expected to replace their infusion sites every 2-3 days – this consists of refilling the pump reservoir, rewinding/repriming the pump and tubing, and inserting a completely new subcutaneous cannula site. This is not an expressly "private" process – save for perhaps the cannula reinsertion component – and surrounding persons are usually intermittently aware. Second, the pump, although generally covered by strategically located personal garments or accessories, is not completely invisible, and should at least make a cameo during mealtimes. Many diabulimia patients exhibit a noticeable deficiency of the pump in bodily vicinity, either having disconnected or suspended it for extended periods of time. Unless the pump is on a "vibrate" setting for alarms or notifications, observers might hear constant staccato beeping which derives from any of the following: a perpetual "suspend" setting, low battery, necessity for maintenance or refilling/repriming, and emergency shutoff after remaining untouched for a preset period of time (safety mechanism). These alarms are easily rectified, and their persistence indicates misuse.

One pump is relatively less vulnerable to manipulation than others, and is also useful for closely monitoring insulin adherence (no average feat considering the pump dynamic): a more recent model labeled the Omnipod™. Marketed primarily as a 'tubeless' pump, it consists basically of two sets of mechanics. The first is the "pod," which is connected subcutaneously to the patient as in any other pump system, and contains adjoined insulin delivery machinery. This apparatus communicates wirelessly with the "Personal Diabetes Manager," a.k.a. the PDM: a 'remote control' that the patient must use to instruct the pod regarding relevant blood glucose values, correction factors, and insulin boluses. The PDM is also utilized during routine cannula insertion, which is an essentially 'needle–less' process: the patient removes the pod from the packaging, fills the reservoir with insulin, and attaches the entire apparatus to the skin via adhesive. After completing these steps, the patient (via the PDM) instructs the pod to 'insert the cannula.' The process is accomplished completely internally under the pod's encapsulation, with an auto-withdraw mechanism for the needle. This system is virtually unique for the Omnipod, as it never exposes the patient to the cannula needle. Also, because it eliminates the ability to detach tubing from a stably fixed cannula site, which is executed autonomously to sever the source of exogenous insulin, the only ways to forego a programmed dose are to 1.) remove the pod or cannula, or 2.) fail to attach or insert them at all. Doctoring boluses and basal rates is consequently more difficult. In general, the features of fewer accessible components make the Omnipod relatively less susceptible to subterfuge. Another feature ideal for the purposes of recognition is the rather bulky profile of the pod itself – due to the auxiliary encapsulated machinery, the apparatus creates a sometimes conspicuous ~2x3inch protrusion which should usually be perceptible, or at least presentable upon request (recent release of smaller pods has rendered this manner of detection less feasible). For this reason, the Omnipod is sometimes used in inpatient rehabilitation centers – physicians can appropriate the PDM and use it as a type of 'remote control' to ensure that the patient receives the prescribed insulin dose.

However, the Omnipod is also not infallible in terms of its vulnerability towards manipulation. In regards to inpatient treatment, it is logistically impossible for the endocrinologist to attend all meals, and due to lack of training nurses cannot administer insulin via the PDM. Hence, the only feasible alternative is relinquishing the PDM to the patient, thus granting them a minimal but adequate window of time to manipulate their dose without supervision. The outpatient discussion concerns more the non-autonomous population for whom there is an adult monitor, as there is no long-term benefit for the rigmarole of 'pod appearance' if another party is not keeping vigil. The important mechanical principle here is such: the 'pod' and the 'cannula' cannot be regarded as a single entity. That is to say, apparent attachment of the pod does not entail concomitant insertion of the cannula. It is possible to dispatch the cannula either 1.) directly into the skin, then remove the entire pod with the cannula and reposition the adhesive onto the skin, or 2.) into air prior to applying the pod to the skin, such that the cannula is exposed beforehand. In both cases, the end result is that the cannula is simply left to lie apposed to the bare skin (rather than *under* it). Kinking of the cannula is usually an impediment to these methods (in which circumstance the PDM will alert and curtail insulin administration until the situation is rectified).

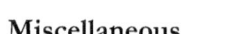

Miscellaneous

- ### *Diabetes Supplies*

Another sign is progressive accumulation of insulin and pump equipment, which signifies that the patient is employing components of their insulin regimen at a frequency alarmingly less than what their physician has recommended (if the supplies are being ordered/filled as per prescription instructions). Families have testified that insulin vials will pile up in the fridge, boxes of infusion sets and pump reservoirs collect dust for years, and syringes remain untouched until they spill out from the cabinetry. Alternatively, the patient might deny the need for prescription refills (a more useful sign if another family member is ordering medications).

- *Ketones*

Although not part of a diabetic patient's daily schedule, and indeed, usually used only sporadically (to ensure absence in the face of elevated blood glucose readings), ketone testing might prove elucidative as well. Refusal to, or skittishness associated with, the testing of ketones should arouse some misgivings. Unfortunately, this avenue's ceiling of utility caps at soliciting the PWDb's response to measuring their ketones, as the veracity of testing is mechanistically difficult to validate. The procedure requires holding a narrow diagnostic strip directly under a stream of urine or inside a receptacle where a fresh urine sample has been deposited. Unfortunately, there is no plausible means to ensure that the urine sample has not been adulterated. The PWDb might dilute the aliquot with tap or toilet bowl water, thus logarithmically underestimating the amount of ketones present.

- *Eating Habits*

Secretive eating patterns is a more qualitative nuance. This symptom might be relatively more difficult to observe with restrictive PWDbs (consumption is drastically reduced, leaving little substance to hide; whatever minutiae the patient permits themselves to eat, however, is usually in private.) On the other hand, if the patient is of the bingeing subtype, they might buy large amounts of "diabetes-forbidden" fare such as sugary, subnutritious foods/drinks, and consume them in private. Some might notice this as a "hoarding" of quantities far in excess of what others would regard as appropriate. Their intake of food in public might be standard, above/below normal, so this is not usually an accurate barometer concerning existence of an eating disorder. Families might find that their pantry provisions are exhausted in inordinate amounts of time without knowing precisely their allocation.

Long-term Deception

The main person to convince on a longitudinal timescale is the treating endocrinologist (or primary care physician, nurse practitioner, and such). Failure leaves the patient at risk for highly undesirable outcomes: 1.) disclosure to the parent or guardian of the adverse behaviors (if the patient is under 18), and/or 2.) referral to a mental health professional for depression/insulin noncompliance issues, or 3.) recognition of an insulin-omitting eating disorder and subsequent intervention (if the endocrinologist is so equipped), and 4.) perceived stigma – even if no intervention is anticipated, patients still feel profound shame and guilt knowing that other people are aware of their actions. The clinician should be at least marginally convinced of the PWDb's "adherence" so to avoid such consequences. (Whether or not the endocrinologist realizes the true psychopathology is a completely different issue, and involves a crucial distinction between the physical act of manipulating insulin and the underlying cognitive displacement. It is easier to determine that a patient is not taking insulin than it is to realize that this is prompted by an intentional and pathological effort to control weight.)

Depending on the patient's diabetes control, an endocrinologist generally recommends clinic appointments every 2-5 months. One essential feature of these routine appointments is obtaining the glycosylated hemoglobin value (abbreviated as the HbA1c, or A1c). This is a measure of the patient's approximate average blood glucose level, and is a quantitative aid for the physician in determining how well the patient has controlled their diabetes for 2-3 months prior to the visit. It can be obtained from either 1.) whole blood/serum (generally ordered by/drawn prior to the appointment by the primary care physician, for patients who need other lab values tested concomitantly, e.g. lipid panels, electrolytes, thyroid function, and such; alternatively the endocrinologist can also order independently), or 2.) point-of-care testing (POCT), which is determined directly in the endocrinologist's office.

The foundation of the HbA1c is the reaction of glucose with the hemoglobin abundant in red blood cells, which (through a series of *reversible* intermediates) irreversibly forms a glycated hemoglobin molecule. (Many different physiological proteins form covalent linkages with glucose, but hemoglobin is the substance of quantitative choice for this diagnostic purpose, due to its high natural concentration in red blood cells.) When the concentration of glucose is increased, as is the consequence of insulin omission, both the quantity and rate of formation of this molecule are also increased.[9]

---

[9] It is useful to know the governing kinetics of the sequence of reactions between glucose and hemoglobin. This elucidates many of the problems inherent to this diagnostic, especially in the light of potential deception and discrepancy due to the diabulimic pattern of insulin omission (restrictive or binging), as well as the trio of variables (frequency, amplitude, and duration, as presented in Chapter 3).

1.)The formation of the glycosylated hemoglobin molecule (aka HbA1c), is a two step, non-enzymatic (spontaneous) reaction.[2] First, the aldehyde functional group of the glucose molecule rapidly and reversibly reacts with the -NH_2 terminal of the hemoglobin chain to form an aldimine (also known as a Schiff base) intermediate. (Although the glucose aldehyde can react with many sites on the hemoglobin molecule, the -NH_2 terminal is the most common, most rapid, and roughly reflective of the total HbA1c in erythrocytes.) [3]

The forward step is rate-limiting and second order, proportional to the concentrations of hemoglobin ([H]) and glucose ([G]): $Rate_{aldimine} = k_1[H][G]$. k_1 is the forward rate constant, which has been experimentally determined to be 0.9 $mM^{-1}hr^{-1}$. The reverse step – dissociation of the intermediate aldimine into glucose and hemoglobin, is first order, proportional to the concentration of the aldimine ([H=G]): $Rate_{glucose+hemoglobin} = K_{-1}[H=G]$. K_{-1} is the reverse rate constant, which has been experimentally determined to be 0.35 h^{-1} (about a third the rate of the forward reaction).

2.) Next, the intermediate aldimine Schiff base slowly and irreversibly forms the final ketoamine product, aka the glycosylated HbA1c molecule. This reaction is first order and depends on the concentration of the aldimine intermediate ([H=G]): $Rate_{ketoamine} = K_2[H=G]$. K_2 is likewise the forward rate constant and has been experimentally determined to be 0.0055 h^{-1} (This is roughly one-sixtieth the rate of the K_{-1}, the reverse reaction from H=G to H + G.)

$$
\begin{array}{ccc}
\text{HC=O} & \text{HC=N-}\beta\text{A} & \text{CH}_2\text{-NH}_2^+\beta\text{A} \\
| & | & | \\
\text{HCOH} & \text{HCOH} & \text{C=O} \\
| & | & | \\
\beta\text{-NH}_2 \;+\; \text{HOCH} & \xrightarrow[k_{-1}]{k_1} \;\text{HOCH} & \xrightarrow{k_2}\; \text{HOCH} \\
\boxed{\text{HbA}} \quad | & | & | \\
\text{HCOH} & \text{HCOH} & \text{HCOH} \\
| & | & | \\
\text{HCOH} & \text{HCOH} & \text{HCOH} \\
| & | & | \\
\text{CH}_2\text{OH} & \text{CH}_2\text{OH} & \text{CH}_2\text{OH} \\[4pt]
\boxed{\text{Glucose}} & \boxed{\begin{array}{c}\text{Aldimine}\\\text{Pre-A1c}\end{array}} & \boxed{\begin{array}{c}\text{Ketoamine}\\\text{HbA1c}\end{array}}
\end{array}
$$

Figure 1: *Adapted from Higgins et al. (1981)*[1]

The values of each of the rate constants here are important for the interpretation of the HbA1c value as pertaining to the PWDb. First of all, because K_{-1} is much greater in value than K_2, and the rate of the reverse reaction is dependent on the concentration of H=G, the pool of available H=G will accumulate to a certain level and subsequently plateau – having attained chemical equilibrium. Therefore, when the blood sugar is normalized even for a short amount of time, the Schiff aldimine intermediate will embrace the opportunity to convert back to glucose and hemoglobin, depleting the pool of intermediate aldimine and thus the overall accumulation of final glycated ketoamine. (Indeed, researchers have attributed the conspicuous decrease in HbA1c upon return to proper metabolic control to the depleted pool of aldimine intermediate.[1]) Likewise, if the blood sugar spikes temporarily but inordinately high, the levels of intermediate will climb in parallel, and will more rapidly be converted back to glucose + hemoglobin than they will form the final glycated product. Both instances represent a failure of steady-state. As the attainment of equilibrium favors the final formation of the glycated product, failure to achieve this chemical state secondary to rapidly changing blood glucose levels will tend to underestimate the true average value of the blood glucose levels.

Valleys of euglycemia and spikes of hyperglycemia are both characteristic of diabulimia. Whether or not the PWDb displays symptoms of "restricting" or "bingeing," they might alternate between periods of omission and compliance. These acute periods of hyperglycemia, particularly relevant for binge-eaters, might successfully be concealed by periods during which the PWDb is completely or at least marginally compliant – this sequence might be pre-calculated, or completely unanticipated. Whether the above discussion is will result in clinically distinguishable values and subsequent management modification is another issue altogether.

Another important point is that the HbA1c is an average value, which automatically implies that any outstanding episodes of hyperglycemia might be

The POCT test is painless and very similar to checking a blood glucose level. A finger prick and application of a miniscule amount of blood to the tip of a capillary tube is all that is required. A larger transducer dock performs either chromatography or immunoassay on the sample, and the HbA1c is calculated in as few as three minutes.

The 'tone' of the visit is set by the glycosylated hemoglobin value – when within range (or comparable to those of previous clinic visits), the appointment subsequently consists of prescription updates, cursory review of system questions, and physical examination of feet, eyes, fingertips, and injection sites. If the value is out of range, the endocrinologist will discuss plans by which the patient might improve their glucose control – e.g. through dietary modification, more frequent blood testing; alternatively they might put the patient on a different type of or increased insulin regimen. However, due to the mechanistic stipulations surrounding this value (some of which are discussed in the footnote, making it at times slightly unreliable) physicians might cross-reference the patient's blood sugar monitor as well as insulin pump (if one is used). This aids in determining diurnal trends in blood sugars not expressly revealed by the HbA1c. An HbA1c of 6% corresponds to an average glucose level of 125 (and 28 mg/dl for every 1% in HbA1c above), and clinical antennae must be raised if these two levels are more than appreciably disparate.

Given the above outline of a standard endocrinologist checkup, the patient with diabulimia finds ways to avoid their physician discovering that they are not taking proper levels of insulin. One of the most fruitful ways of accomplishing this is simply by neglecting to see the physician. Records will show gaps of months, even years, between visits. The patient of any age

---

blunted by similar periods of hypoglycemia (to an extent, given the reactions described above). Therefore, if a PWDb omits insulin for a binging episode followed by strict metabolic control for a period of time, it will likely not register in the A1c value. Furthermore, the HbA1c is a weighted average, in that 50% of the level was determined by the plasma glucose value in the month prior to measurement, 25% by the month preceding the first, and likewise 25% in the third month past. Any transgressions committed during the earlier periods preceding an endocrinologist visit are disproportionately represented in the glycated hemoglobin value, contributing to misrecognition of insulin omission if the patient has maintained relatively acceptable metabolic control for the recent past, as they often do in 'preparation' for a clinic appointment.[5-6]

might have multiple no-shows, effect a charade of setting appointments and then canceling them prematurely, or give paltry excuses shortly before the clinic date. Whatever the technique, the purpose plainly boils down to less net time at the clinic, less opportunity for the physician to observe/question their diabetes regimen, and a maintained masquerade.

There are means by which the POCT HbA1c process might be overridden as well, but these are quite involved. As this "level" is expressed as a percentage of A1c hemoglobin molecules that are glycosylated, analogous methods of duping blood sugar monitors such as dilution with external liquids will not affect the readout. Likewise, complete substitution of other substances is futile, as the value being analyzed consists of a physiological molecule (hemoglobin) not easily replicated or produced by an external source as compared to glucose. The same specious mediums such as calibration liquids or saliva cannot be used even though the physical process of obtaining the value is quite similar. Although it seems ludicrous (and nigh obsessive), the nurse/personnel doing the prep work *must* perform all steps themselves, leaving nothing to the patient (sometimes, for comfort, the patient is allowed to prick their own finger with their own lancet in order to obtain the blood sample, which must *not* be allowed). Patients have been caught transferring other peoples' (or even animals') blood to replace their own. It is said that desperation is the mother of invention, and accordingly there are generally no reservations in crossing ordinary boundaries to achieve any one of these ends.

As mentioned above, a diabetes clinician will usually not rely solely on the HbA1c, but will also refer to the timeline of values present in the glucose testing kit and insulin pump (if used). Unfortunately, the glycosylated hemoglobin might be the only assessment available, e.g. the patient has "forgotten to bring" their insulin pump or glucose testing kit, which is also doubtful. Another simple screening tool is checking the meter for current date/time accuracy – sometimes the insouciant PWDb will have attained such levels of disinterest that they do not bother ensuring the accuracy of these values.

The patient will also attempt to rehash the values obtained from these devices. (There are many types of insulin pumps on the market featuring different perks, programs, 'wizards,' calculators, and analyses; however, there are certain components common to all pumps which may be manipulated, and these are what we outline here.) The meticulous patient will have maintained a suitable level of deception pertaining to their glucose monitors and insulin pumps, giving themselves fake 'boluses' that register on the pump and therefore on the readout that the physician obtains upon checkup. This is difficult to perpetuate, however, and the patterns of insulin administration given this method will more often than not appear highly irregular. Basal rates might sporadically be doctored without proper justification. Infusion sets, usually reprimed every 2-3 days, will appear on the readout as occurring at extended or irregular intervals. Looking at the 'alert history' in the pump archives will reveal recalcitrant 'no delivery,' 'no power,' and 'low battery,' alarms.

Sometimes, the patient might attempt to effect a 'time travel' if they are particularly inspired. It is possible to iteratively change the time/date of the pump/glucose monitor to one in the recent past, then administer a fake bolus or sugar reading. The time/date is doctored again, and the same process repeated, such that a rather elegant history is constructed. This 'time travel' is difficult to detect with glucose kits, but in insulin pumps there are two glaring and insurmountable problems. The first involves the basal insulin rate. If a period of three months is being reinvented over the course of a few hours (or however long the patient requires to manually craft the time travel) the basal rate will not register at all. The end result is then a series of counterfeit boluses minus the prescribed basal rate(s). The second problem, albeit very nonspecific, is that the phony boluses will not match the blood sugar readings on the readouts, in both temporal as well as proper dose magnitude. The most salient indication of spurious readouts is their overall imperfection, being riddled with nonsensical hiatuses and odd spikes of insulin dosing.

As reiterated, this level of fastidiousness is not commonly observed. The key intimations are 1.) periods of prolonged pump suspension, 2.) vast deficiency in appropriate pump activity, and 3.) incongruous and inconsistent dosing. These indicate periods during which the patient failed (most likely purposefully) to take proper amounts of insulin.

Towards Recognition

In some clinical settings, the patient provides a 'logbook' along with the glucose meter. Here, each glucose value is recorded by hand as they are measured, in a pocket-sized journal that provides a convenient home readout and eliminates the need to traverse through the meter's archive. Before electronic glucometer readouts largely replaced their utilization in the clinic, these logbooks were the only resource with which the endocrinologist could obtain an overall gestalt of the patient's glucose trends. They are still useful for this purpose if there is a technical difficulty with the glucometer, or if the patient uses multiple testing devices (one for home, car, work, etc.), and such. Suspicion must be aroused, however, when 1.) the logbook is offered expressly in lieu of the glucometer, 2.) the average readings in the logbook do not correspond to the HbA1c level as described above, and/or 3.) the numbers are immaculately written in what appears to be the same pen and similar inflection of handwriting, as if they were transcribed (i.e. "invented") simultaneously.

In addressing blood glucose monitors and the clinical appointment, we must briefly return to reconnoiter the CGM. Although there is minimal anecdotal evidence with regards to diabulimic manipulation given its relatively recent integration within the diabetes market, there are a few warning signs upon the readouts/downloads that should inspire a few qualms and elicit further evaluation. As mentioned, an autonomous patient will most likely completely forego use of this device due to its recalcitrance concerning doctoring; as such this discussion is most relevant for patients 1.) under parental monitoring, and 2.) endeavoring self-treatment for diabulimia recovery, who will intermittently demonstrate stringent compliance with their diabetes regimen, and at other times eliminate it completely (and the intervening spectrum therein).

The CGM software transposes its accumulated data to a line graph plotted as time of day vs. blood glucose. At times, the pump and the CGM cannot communicate with each other, the most common etiology of which involves proximity (sensor/transmitter placed too far away from pump, less static electricity discharge and calibration errors). This is represented on the electronic readout as a 'break' in the continuous line plot. While these hiatuses might periodically be expected (e.g. when the patient changes the sensor, takes a shower, goes swimming, or any activity requiring greater than 40 minutes of separation), the frequency should be no greater than a few times in a short interval, and the duration should not be greater than a few hours. Deviations above these allowances are suspicious – the patient might purposefully be hindering this correspondence if they want to prevent documentation of elevated glucose (as will be present 1.) during a period of insulin restriction, and/or 2.) post-binge with or without restriction). There might be days sans pump-sensor communication, during which the patient will also demonstrate minimal pump activity (e.g. bolusing, basal administration, priming, and such).

References:
1.) Higgins, P., and H. Bunn. "Kinetic Analysis of the Nonenzymatic Glycosylation of Hemoglobin." *Journal of Clinical Investigation 57 (1981): 1652-659.*
2.) Bunn, H. F., D. N. Haney, S. Kamin, K. H. Gabbay, and P. M. Gallop. "The Biosynthesis of Human Hemoglobin A1c. Slow Glycosylation of Hemoglobin in Vivo." *Journal of Clinical Investigation 57.6 (1976): 1652-659.*
3.) Bunn, H., D. Haney, K. Gabbay, and P. Gallop. "Further Identification of the Nature and Linkage of the Carbohydrate in Hemoglobin A1c." *Biochemical and Biophysical Research Communications 67.1 (1975).*
4.) Shih, Grace. DIABULIMIA: *Diabetes + Eating Disorders; What It Is and How to Treat It: A Guide for Individuals and Families.* N.p.: CreateSpace Independent Platform, 2011. Print.
5.) Takara, Y., K. Shima. "The Response of GHb to stepwise plasma glucose change over time in diabetic patients. *Diabetes Care 16: 1313-1314, 1993.*
6.) Tahara, Y., and K. Shima. "Kinetics of HbA1c, Glycated Albumin, and Fructosamine and Analysis of Their Weight Functions against Preceding Plasma Glucose Level."*Diabetes Care 18.4 (1995): 440-47.*
7.) Ruedy, Katrina, and William Tamborlane. "The Landmark JDRF Continuous Glucose Monitoring Randomized Trials: A Look Back at the Accumulated Evidence."*Journal of Cardiovascular Translational Research 5 (2012): 380-87. Print.*

Towards Recognition

CHAPTER 6

SCREENING
AND
PREVENTION

I watched them. I watched them all, like a vicious falcon watches over her dribbling chicks, like a tax collector and his edifices of gold. I watched them as they watched me, let them think they were one step ahead, one hop-skip-and-a-jump in front of me and my agenda and my elaborate theatre of fraud. Did they even care to know better?

"You must feel horribly sick every day, don't you?" one of my doctors asked accusingly after seeing my HbA1c level. I do, but I'm standing up, aren't I, I'm walking, speaking coherently, loving, hating, and living? What do you know? I know what you think — that it's going to catch up with me one of these days, that it was already snapping nastily at my heels. You think I can just start sticking needles into my skin and numbers into my pump, lancets into my fingertips and rabbit greens onto my plate, and patch the pieces of my derailed life back together?

Some days I wanted to tell them. I wanted to show them everything I had done, tell them that they were wrong, that I had cheated science and physiology and biochemistry and medicine and consequence and philosophy, that I was so resilient my body could survive without insulin for so long and not endure any of what they had threatened. I had won and they had lost. I desperately wanted to let slip some subtle intimation that this was, in fact, what had happened, what I was capable of sustaining.

But even that would be a lie. I didn't want them to know that I was able to outmaneuver them. Because I wanted them to be smarter. I wanted them to show me they could fix me. I wanted them to recognize that I was the injured one here, that they shouldn't be standing on the other side of the examining table with my parents, my insulin vials, my dusty glucose monitor, condemning, indicting, prosecuting…

Very well, I'm the sinner; you can have that. But it's not supposed to be me against you. And you, and you. That's not the way this is supposed to work.

Towards Recognition

Insulin-dependent diabetes mellitus, while obviously a challenge for the patient, is likewise not simple for the clinician to treat. It does not entail a static prescription or necessarily predictable conclusions. The sine qua non of Type I diabetes is mutual education of both patient and physician, a certain level of clinical vigilance for positive outcomes, and instances of frustration and disillusionment. Within the space of one time-constrained clinical appointment, the endocrinologist must survey and possibly calibrate a multitude of variables: previous history, lab values, hemoglobin A1c, patient demeanor, daily blood glucose and insulin dosing patterns, frequency of hypoglycemic episodes, prescriptions, insulin pump modifications, basal/bolus rates, sensors, dietary profile, focused physical exam – all while attempting to communicate directly with the patient in as productive and personable a fashion so to distill all pertinent information. And when this patient is expressly resentful or frightened of the entire clinical environment (as is generally the case with a PWDb), any lack of physician alertness might result in acute loss of useful diagnostic information.

In the endeavor to flush out a putative case of diabulimia, the endocrinologist (or primary care doctor, nurse practitioner, physician's assistant, certified diabetes educator) is typically thwarted on multiple fronts. They have very little opportunity to screen for an eating disorder, let alone determine whether said disorder involves intentional insulin omission. First of all, they must actually 1.) discern the potential for and 2.) recognize that the patient is displaying classic symptoms of disturbed eating (through a variety of tactful screening questions/questionnaires). Second, the clinician must then inquire as to whether the patient is using insulin as a way to control their weight without soliciting a defensive attitude or 'teaching' them the methodology if it is not the problem. In a vast majority of cases, the patient will more often than not deny outright such an absolutely preposterous idea. Next, if through a Herculean effort extended through perhaps multiple clinic visits and carefully crafted queries, the clinician finally manages to coerce or flush out the pathology, they might not even possess the knowledge of how to address the illness nor to whom the patient should be referred. This ultimate impasse can even preclude initiating the line of questioning – why attempt to unearth a condition when the resources with which to treat it are inaccessible? This is yet regrettably the situation for many patients and their diabetes teams.

There is a spectrum of diabulimia recognition across the clinical realm, which fortunately has increased overall in recent years. Mental health professionals specializing in eating disorders (by virtue of their professions) may be cognizant of its existence as a purging mechanism in anorexia nervosa or bulimia nervosa – although perhaps not always under the label of "diabulimia" but rather 'insulin omission' or a phrase to the same effect. Primary care physicians and endocrinologists, on the other hand, are not explicitly trained in the symptomatic presentation of eating disorders. They are generally poised to dismiss the signs of diabulimia as non-adherence or innocent difficulty to control blood sugar, given the lack of a "rational" umbrella. While it is true that mental health professionals can be consulted by the patient before anyone else in the healthcare sequence, it is highly unlikely that Type I diabetic patients, especially those with eating disorders, will visit them directly (i.e. sans referral, recommendation, or even coercion). This is testament to the innate nature of eating disorders – patients are either in denial of their condition, or recognize its presence but do not want to relinquish control to the treatment process. As such, voluntarily committing themselves firsthand to the care of a mental health professional is fundamentally counterproductive. Unless the patient is underage (where parents/guardians might exercise authority to bring them to a mental health clinic if they recognize certain symptoms), this probability is quite slim. Diabulimia patients are also sometimes unable to visit a mental health clinician secondary to hierarchic convolutions of the healthcare system: depending on the patient's specific coverage, referrals from a primary care physician or endocrinologist might be required. Other factors involve impediments and ignominy (cultural or otherwise) surrounding contact with the mental health specialty (which has actually tapered in recent years). Parents/guardians are also, perhaps counterintuitively, a powerful hindrance to diabulimia recognition in some cases. Some simply cannot internalize the concept that their child is suffering from an eating disorder, let alone abusing insulin as an executive mechanism. Occasionally, the stigma of association with the psychiatric realm is no less potent for the parent than it is for the patient, due to implications concerning the guardians themselves. Nuclear relatives might feel that such a suggestion is a flagrant insult to their methods of upbringing – an affront to their integrity or that of their child. Whatever the etiology, many parents will ignore recommendations to – indeed, take proactive stances *against* – bring their child to a mental health professional.

As such, the people optimally equipped to address diabulimia are not first in the line of clinical sight. This is obviously a significant detriment to patients of all ages. For pre-adolescents and adolescents, a lack of recognition on the part of the endocrinologist might totally preclude any recommendation to a mental health professional – deception and denial often successfully conceal any clue of an underlying disorder. Parents/guardians consequently neglect to follow up with the physician who actually might diagnose and treat their child's disturbed eating. For older and autonomous patients (e.g. young adults), visiting a clinician ill-equipped with the skills and knowledge essential to recognize the condition will only serve to reinforce their sense of autonomy over abnormal behavioral patterns. Such an encounter might also cement their disillusionment towards the medical system's ability to help their condition, considering the primary misrecognition. These entrenched perceptions project to further thwart any mental health interventions.

As discussed in Chapter 2, the denomination of ED-DMT1 (Eating Disorders – Diabetes Mellitus Type I) is a significant step towards enhancing physician awareness of insulin omission as a technique for weight control. Given the recent propagation of consciousness regarding this significant medical issue, more doctors (endocrinologists especially) are starting to recognize that diabetes and eating disorders/insulin manipulation (especially within certain demographics) frequently walk in tandem. The last, and perhaps most recalcitrant, deficit to be reconciled is between knowledge and practice – even if physicians are aware of diabulimia in theory, the ability to distinguish it in reality is a completely different matter. As such, not only must they know the heralds of such pathologies but also execute certain techniques to more comprehensively expose their existence. These procedures include either/both 1.) diplomatic questioning, which currently integrates well within the standard patient appointment, and 2.) administration of diabetes-specific screening questionnaires to patients within the appropriate demographic and/or with a suspicious past medical history (i.e. those with a high pretest probability). The latter needs further mechanistic development within the present clinical dynamic, but it is a solid template with which physicians can possibly perceive patients with diabulimia/ED-DMT1.

Differential Diagnosis

The differential diagnosis for the more familiar presenting symptoms of diabulimia encompasses a multitude of pathologies. (Here, we cannot ignore that "diabulimia" codifies patients suffering from either anorexia nervosa ['restrictive' diabulimia subtype] or bulimia nervosa ['bingeing' diabulimia subtype]. As such, they are included in the differential below. The following are not ranked in order of likelihood; many are comorbid with each other. Observable/relayed symptoms (which sometimes overlap with those found in diabulimia) supporting each diagnosis are italicized under the disorder, and may include:

1. Bulimia nervosa
   - *Weight gain/loss, swollen face, lethargy, pallor, fatigue, irregular menstruation, flat affect, slow speech, psychomotor retardation [less common], low self-esteem, may deny eating problem, tachycardia, hypotension, typically elevated A1c*
2. Anorexia nervosa
   - *Weight loss, swollen face, lanugo (fine facial hair), amenorrhea, flat affect, slow speech, psychomotor retardation [less common], low self-esteem, may deny eating problem, denial of weight abnormality, bradycardia, hypotension, typically normal A1c*
3. Noncompliance with diabetes (teenage rebellion, 'burnout,' laxity, forgetfulness)
   - *Hyperglycemia, fatigue, weight change, increased appetite, confusion, altered mental status, may include fear of hypoglycemia, family conflict*
4. Binge-eating disorder
   - *Weight gain, water retention (edema), symptoms of depression/anxiety, elevated A1c*
5. Depression/Mood disorder
   - *Psychomotor agitation/retardation, guilt, fatigue, flat speech/affect, sleep disturbances, appetite changes, weight gain/loss*
6. Drug abuse/misuse (prescribed or otherwise)
   - *Variety*
7. Electrolyte imbalance (intake/excretion/metabolic)

Others: Polycystic ovarian syndrome, Cushing's syndrome/disease, cardiovascular pathology, infection (more commonly respiratory, gastrointestinal, reproductive tract)

Screening Questions

The most logical course of action when assessing a suspicious patient is to determine 1.) whether they are suffering from an eating disorder, then 2.) whether or not they regularly attempt to purge. If both of these are present, then the clinician should determine 3.) whether they are using insulin to effect the purging, and subsequently 4.) whether or not insulin omission is a.) the sole mechanism of purging, b.) ancillary to a more conventional method such as emesis/laxatives, or c.) the principle method supplemented by another. '1' and 'c' have graver implications for metabolic control, as intentional insulin abuse provides a directly deleterious effect on blood sugar. Other purging mechanisms are more circuitous in their detriment but often disturb electrolyte balance. (Of course, all of the above four guidelines assumes that the clinician has the time, resources, and opportunity to pursue such an avenue of questioning. As mentioned above, they are obstructed at several points along this endeavor, which, over and on top of everything, is certainly not as linear as described above.)

Alternatively – and this is the path less traveled – the physician might determine the presence of insulin restriction at the onset. The advantages to this approach include the existence of many clues oftentimes *sensitive* for omission: aberrant HbA1c levels, lack of diabetes activity as evinced by glucose kit and pump readouts, and recurrent hospitalizations for DKA. Given other evidence, such as the patient's age and gender (and years post-diagnosis), the physician can synthesize the clinical presentation into an illustration of diabulimia. However, these symptoms have a lamentable lack of *specificity* – viz., their etiologies can be attributed to pathologies unrelated to weight control – and caution must consequently be exercised when postulating the existence of insulin omission for the purpose of weight control. Many factors may cause insulin omission and may not be related to an underlying eating disorder. However, as eating disorders and insulin manipulation frequently interdigitate, addressing a suspicious patient is more efficiently accomplished through the former approach.

The necessity of tact is *central* to the screening process of a patient suspected to suffer from this illness. There is, first and foremost, a powerful sense of shame surrounding any psychological disorder like diabulimia – especially in the perception of the patient, let alone the people relevant to their daily existence. Also innate to the PWDb are sensations of self-reproach for the perceived inability to control their own actions, or for acting as the agent of destruction to their own bodies. In the words of one 19-year-old girl, *"I read about a boy dying of leukemia today, and I thought to myself – I should be in his place. I was born healthy, I was given a chance to have a normal life even with diabetes. But look what I've done to myself. He deserves life so much more than I do…"* If the clinician fails to comprehend the exquisite delicacy of these situations or if they forego discretion for the candor of frustration, then they risk permanent distrust which obliterates the possibility that the patient will open up to them or anyone else. Patients with diabulimia live in a state of palpable trepidation, where the dread of repercussion for manipulating insulin in the first place meshes with the greater fear that someone else will strong-arm them into therapy.

While speaking to a susceptible patient, then, the clinician should allay any misgivings leading them to believe that they might be steered against their will. The PWDb's attitude towards treatment and recovery (namely, reinstitution of appropriate insulin therapy and dietary management) is often paroxysmally ambivalent. To live with diabulimia is to daily persevere through adverse physical symptoms (exhaustion, indigestion, vomiting, thirst, hunger, urination) which interfere with baseline levels of functioning. While some express a desire for liberation, they cannot reconcile it with the coexistent motivations at the source of their disordered eating behaviors. The physical hindrances of diabulimia, however debilitating, constitute small sacrifices compared with the particular compromises they would have to make during treatment. This is why some take such painstaking care in hiding their condition.

The most useful questions are oblique, those which are inconspicuous and 'casual' enough to be integrated into the average endocrinologist appointment. This type of approach is especially productive when addressing patients who are intentionally specious or wary when addressed concerning their condition. Direct inquiries also have significant utility and can likewise yield enlightening information, but there is a higher risk that the patient will 'clam up' secondary to suspicion, fear, or anxiety. Ordering of questions depends on each patient's particular circumstances and attitudes towards eating, weight, diabetes, and even relationship with the physician. Likewise, an inquiry's utility and its ability to inspire wariness are couched in the clinician's stylistic demeanor and the sequence/manner in which it is incorporated into the interview. (This is obviously an individually cultivated skill.)

The following list enumerates some questions which might prove helpful for screening.[3] A variety might be elected for use, but a positive response does not 'cinch' the diagnosis – integration with previous history, chief complaint, and physical examination findings is essential. For example, the response to "Do you feel frustrated/guilty/overwhelmed when you are unable to control your blood glucose?" will likely be affirmative for a majority of patients, but might lend additional corroboration of the illness. Indeed, many of these are relatively nonspecific, and as such should be tailored with discretion for each individual patient/physician relationship. Asking a few questions per clinical appointment is ideal, rather than foisting the entire gamut in an abbreviated period of time:

- ➤ Do you enjoy the foods that you eat?
- ➤ Do you sometimes feel you have to limit what you eat because you have diabetes?
- ➤ Do you sometimes eat in secret?
- ➤ Do you, on occasion, feel uncontrolled when you eat?
- ➤ Do you sometimes have trouble controlling your blood sugar because your appetite is increased or decreased, or if you eat too much/too little?
- ➤ How frequently do you feel preoccupied with your weight?
- ➤ How often do you weigh yourself? Do you feel frustrated or irritated if/when you gain weight?
- ➤ How much would you like to weigh? Tell me why this is ideal for you.
- ➤ Have you ever tried to lose weight before? What ways do you use to try to lose weight? Do you ever skip meals to lose weight?

- ➤ Do you ever 'go on a diet', and if so, what kind? Do you find it difficult to stay on this diet? Have you been successful? How much weight have you lost and over what period of time?
- ➤ Do you feel that your family/friends scrutinize your weight?
- ➤ Did you start to think about your weight more after you were diagnosed with diabetes and had to take insulin?
- ➤ How much do you weigh? (Asked for purposes of comparison with the actual value measured in the clinic if the patient has not already been notified – useful indicator of perception)
- ➤ Do you feel comfortable with your body or your shape?
- ➤ Are there particular parts of your body with which you feel particularly aware, like your legs or your stomach?
- ➤ Are you able to change in public areas, such as the locker room/swimming pool?
- ➤ Do you ever feel that your diet or your blood sugars have to be perfectly on track? Do you feel frustrated/guilty/angry when they are not?
- ➤ How often do you exercise?
- ➤ Do you sometimes forget to take your insulin?
- ➤ Sometimes, do you just feel like not giving yourself insulin? Is this because you feel frustrated/guilty/overwhelmed/disinterested?
- ➤ How does taking insulin make you feel?
- ➤ Do you think that taking insulin [or any of your other medications] perhaps affects your weight?
- ➤ How regular are your menstrual periods?
- ➤ Have you noticed a decrease in your sex drive lately?
- ➤ Have you ever reached the point or thought of harming yourself?

Clinicians must be sensitive to the possibility of 'advertising' diabulimia during the clinical interview. Although insulin omission for the purpose of weight control is consummately logical, the concept is yet 1.) not expressly evident to a number of patients, or 2.) is evident, but perceived as so completely heinous and self-destructive that further corroboration of its prevalence would be required for actual execution. The physician should exercise caution so as not to inspire *or* validate any likely adverse ideas. For example, painfully candid questions such as "Do you sometimes skip your insulin shots to lose weight?" must be expressly avoided. Even more subtly phrased queries e.g. "How does taking insulin make you feel about your weight?" can inadvertently instill seeds in a susceptible patient.

When the patient is over 18 years of age, physicians are legally constrained by clauses of nondisclosure to parents/guardians, and 'parent-ectomies' are consequently performed prior to the patient interview. However, some clinicians might believe it useful to communicate with or include the parents in the discussion if the patient is underage. Such a setting can facilitate extraction of information that the patient might intentionally or unintentionally be withholding. While this might prove enlightening if executed diplomatically, it also can be interpreted as a breach of trust or crossing of implicit boundaries. Also, some questions such as "Do you eat in secret?" are better asked in situations during which the patient and physician are alone and uninhibited by external influences (or the fear thereof).

The 'HEADS assessment' (acronym for common pubertal issues; the 'E' stands for 'eating disorder,' and the 'S' for suicide, among others), is a well-documented screening tool that can be utilized in a primary care setting to elucidate various lifestyle parameters contributing to a particular pathology. When properly executed, it can help bring diabulimia to light from the onset of presentation to the hierarchical healthcare sequence, thereby expediting assessment and treatment by the appropriate subspecialty. It also assesses the patient's mentation towards suicide, an issue which is highly comorbid with and must be screened for in any patient with an eating disorder.

Questionnaires/Surveys

Opinion differs as to whether there is actually an advantage to the various self-report eating disorder questionnaires in existence, versus the clinical interview discussed above. Presently, eating disorder questionnaires exist only for the general, non-diabetic population – a conspicuous disadvantage which we will discuss further. Arguments in support of the *interview* include the opportunity to explore more complex and specific eating disorders (diabulimia, for example), the interpersonal interaction, and the greater accuracy produced in terms of what the patient interprets as 'bingeing' or 'excessive calories.' Factors favoring the *questionnaire* include elimination of guilt associated with acknowledging certain types of adverse behaviors/beliefs, and the greater veracity/objectivity of the questionnaire self-report given the lack of interpersonal influences. The primary problem with these questionnaires is that they potentially miscalculate the true prevalence of eating disorders in both a population of juvenile diabetics as well as within the individual diabetic patient. Only if pertinent adjustments are instituted, as they relate specifically to patients with Type I diabetes, will these surveys be beneficial to identify disturbed eating behavior. Their contemporary use is essentially in the clinical research field, where standardized methods of administration and more rigorous pooled data analysis render them more viable than 'handing them out while taking the vital signs' during a clinical appointment.

Currently the survey gold standard for identifying patients with eating disorders is the Eating Disorder Examination Questionnaire (EDE-Q)[2] and the child Eating Disorder Examination (chEDE-Q, its modified version for children 8-14 years of age.) This is a 28-question list containing subtle permutations of questions relating to weight, shape, and diet/food. It is designed to determine scores in the areas of excessive dietary restraint, weight concern, eating concern, and shape concern.

One of the main problems with the EDE-Q and other eating disorder questionnaires geared towards the general population is that, quite simply, they are designed for individuals without diabetes. Unfortunately, living (and functioning) with Type I necessitates an above-average degree of knowledge concerning food, diet, nutrition, weight, and calories that – in any other setting – is highly likely to be considered pathological. As such, the use of a completely non-adapted questionnaire such as the EDE-Q for a diabetic patient engenders the risk of overestimating the likelihood of an eating pathology. For example, a question in the EDE-Q inquires as to whether "thinking about food, eating, or calories made it very difficult to concentrate on things you are interested in (for example, working, following a conversation, or reading)?" Another asks "Have you had a definite fear of losing control over eating?" Both of these questions are delegated answer choices of 'No days,' 'Everyday,' '1-5 days,' etc., *ad* 28 days. The answer from a normal, non-eating-disordered diabetic patient would be markedly and quantitatively increased compared to a normal member of the general population. This is perfectly reasonable (and even necessary for a conscientious diabetic lifestyle), given the daily carbohydrate and caloric calculations, social engagements, titrations, and modifications that diabetic patients must incessantly consider. However, if a non-diabetic individual were to report the same magnitude of perseverance for these questions, any clinician would feasibly be concerned about the presence of an eating disorder.

Conversely, the EDE-Q and other questionnaires might possibly *underestimate* the prevalence of eating disorders *within* diabetic populations and individuals. The conventional questionnaires only incorporate vomiting, laxatives, and compulsive/excessive exercise, but by default cannot contain insulin omission. (Non-diabetic patients, by definition, autonomously produce and utilize this molecule, and so restricting or manipulating it is obviously not a feasible purging mechanism.) The underestimation of incidence as well as severity would apply to an eating-disordered patient who is using solely insulin restriction, or insulin restriction in combination with other purging behaviors.

To address these stipulations, Markowitz et al.[1] revised a novel diabetes-specific eating disorder questionnaire, labeled the Diabetes Eating Problem Survey (DEPS). They have confirmed in one study population its internal consistency as well as external validity. Some of the questions are so precise that only a diabetic patient is capable of answering: "I eat to the point of spilling ketones in my urine," "I feel fat when I take all of my insulin," and "When I overeat, I don't take enough insulin to cover the food." Although succinct and candid, this survey has not been shown to adequately address underpinnings of body dysmorphia.

Another study by d'Emden et al.[4] added diabetes/insulin omission-specific questions to two clinical surveys: 1.) the Youth Eating Disorder Examination questionnaire (abbreviated as YEDE-Q, another modified version of the EDE-Q for adolescents), and 2.) the Eating Disorder Inventory-3 Risk Composite (EDI-3RC) and correlated them with the chEDE-Q. Both tailored questionnaires showed high internal consistency and concurrent validity. Although further clinical investigation is warranted, these surveys and their derivatives are slated for implementation in ED-DMT1 and diabulimia.[1]

Some might question the utility of promoting diabulimia recognition due to the lack of both 1.) resources with which to treat the condition even after it is realized, and 2.) interest towards recuperation from the patients themselves. Why flush out diabulimia when you cannot address it, and why address it when the uncooperative patient will only stifle their own treatment? But this rationale represents a ubiquitous impediment to progress – although a valid inquiry, it does not lend fair room for sequential progress. Diabulimia recognition, treatment, and prevention are all in nascent phases of development, and such hindrances do not present insurmountable odds.

If the physician *is* convinced that the patient suffers from an insulin-omitting eating disorder, they are faced with a few choices – not the least of which is to ignore or deny it completely, and treat as they would any other refractory hyperglycemic patient. Unfortunately, for the aforementioned reasons, this is precisely what occurs in a pronounced number of cases – although we cannot conscionably place blame on the patient *or* the clinician. Both are victims of the medical system's gross lack of material (and desire for material) pertaining to diabulimia. Prescribing more insulin, suggesting dietary modifications, chiding the patient for non-adherence, using 'fright' tactics to elicit compliance, ordering unnecessary batteries of diagnostic testing: all of these displace the outstanding issue at hand.

As such, the most useful course of action (regardless of the patient's age) is to refer them to a mental health professional or eating disorder specialist willing to collaborate with the endocrinologist (to better understand Type I if he/she does not already). Recommending/referring to a dietician or nutritionist is also beneficial, but as the underlying problem is psychological, prompt intervention through this avenue is by far the most expedient strategy. Patients will, however, eschew such advice for many reasons – denial and the stigma of psychiatric disorders (witnessed especially with parents of young adolescents), insurance stipulations, prior negative experience with a psychiatrist/psychologist, and desire to protract the illness. In such instances, there is little the clinician can do but lend subtle counsel and wait until the patient is marginally amenable to psychological intervention. They might themselves attempt to provide a rudimentary platform towards this end.

Towards Recognition

It is exquisitely disheartening for the endocrinologist to know that despite their assessments and management efforts, the patient will likely leave their clinic, further perpetuate adverse insulin practices, and progress to salient end-organ damage. Despite these discouraging prospects, it is in the PWDb's best interest for the physician to remain unobtrusive, allow them to make decisions for themselves, and trust that gentle clinical counsel will eventually crystallize. This is an admittedly dissatisfying recommendation, but perhaps the only one that has consistently demonstrated good prognosis.

Prevention

The paradigm of primary prevention dictates that we address the issue of prophylaxis against the development of diabulimia: the "apple a day" that keeps the eating disorder away. This preventative approach can mitigate many of the complications associated with the comorbidity. Although there are very few clinical studies examining methods by which intentional insulin omission might be subverted prior to its first manifestation, this is *not* an uphill battle.

It is more useful here to address impedance of the eating disorder rather than impedance of 'insulin manipulation for the purpose of weight control;' as the chronology of the former is more encapsulative. Research has demonstrated that targeting variables such as self-esteem, media literacy, perfectionism, and dieting are effective in reducing the risk factors associated with disordered eating (although these studies did not specifically examine diabetic populations).

Anecdotally, we cannot further underscore the power of self-esteem – compromising this entity is considered core to the development of disordered eating, and sources multifactorially. Patients with Type I already must traverse life different from their peers in many biosociocultural regards secondary to the chronic illness. Some patients even feel marginally ostracized. Self-esteem is one of the many nuances rendered quite friable, and as such normalizing, strengthening, and reinforcing it from the earliest viable stages is crucial. Internal as well as external validations are both essential, as insult to one jeopardizes integrity of the other. Patients should seek to cultivate productive relationships, learn positive methods by which to address stress (acute and chronic), avoid internalizing criticism, and learn to accept themselves overall. Indeed, non-diabetic low-risk (for eating disorders) adolescents who underwent an interactive, self-esteem education program demonstrated improved scores on body satisfaction; high-risk adolescents likewise demonstrated lower drive for thinness and greater body satisfaction.[6]

One intuitive intervention is didactically founded, in which subjects are taught about eating disorders and any pertinent auxiliary information. Although this approach enhances cognizance of the condition and thereby institutes some protective effects in certain subjects, it also might potentially be harmful in others. In fact, this information-based strategy has consistently been demonstrated in multiple randomized controlled trials to be ineffective towards prevention. It provides 'gratuitous' education that conceivably might never have been encountered by the patient in the first place – increased awareness of their own body image, how to utilize inappropriate compensatory behaviors, and 'pathologizing' of actions which at baseline were likely totally innocuous. As described earlier in the chapter, this advertising effect is especially dangerous for Type I diabetic patients, as it might inadvertently alert already susceptible subjects to the concept of diabulimia, or even validate it by virtue of the knowledge that other patients have both abstracted and actualized the method. In contrast, an interactive approach towards prevention (undertaken with Type I diabetic girls) demonstrated improved outcomes in multiple dimensions, e.g. self-esteem, diabetes control, and thin-ideal internalization. Researchers, rather than using didactic methods, engaged the subjects in multisession discussions concerning positive/negative aspects of diabetes, stress, media stereotypes, and body image.[5,7] Prompting normal subjects to flush out their own ponderings on such issues 1.) permits the therapist to build upon baseline knowledge rather than inoculating with unsolicited information, 2.) provides positive reinforcement for advantageous underlying cognitions, and 3.) helps normal subjects understand how they can harness their own strengths towards more validating experiences with diabetes and otherwise.

Capitalizing upon protective factors for the diabetic also insulates from eating disorder/diabulimia development. One of the most consistently potent entities on this front is interpersonal relationships, especially with the family (if relevant). This includes maintaining familial proximity and involving them in mealtimes and exercise. The patient should not be prevented from communal eating simply because they must adhere to certain inelastic schedules to which their siblings or parents cannot. From these family-centric experiences – by serving from the same platters and drinking from the same pitchers, the patient also nurtures a sense of normality that might have been jeopardized post-diagnosis. This prevents sensations of isolation, as well as any secretive eating patterns that the patient might develop from prohibition of labeled 'un-diabetic' food. Patients should also seek to maintain and/or find positive relationships – platonic, romantic, familial – and use these to maximize on their baseline levels of confidence, extroversion, and social interdigitation. There is evidence to show that harmonious parental (both maternal and paternal) relationships contribute towards the stability of eating patterns and body image. During the 'teen rebellion' stage – so characteristic that it is common Type I vernacular – parents should engage themselves inasmuch as the patient is comfortable, and avoid antagonism due to criticizing subnormal glucose readings and eating patterns.

The ability to critically appraise the media for its oftentimes deceptive intentions and discern any harmful subliminal messages (termed 'media literacy') should also be fostered as warranted. It is not always realistic to avoid images and commentaries containing food or those glamorizing certain body types – they are fairly ubiquitous and intentioned as such, fomenting the body dysmorphia and adverse dietary patterns which are profound risk factors for disordered eating. A prophylactic approach on the media internalization front (akin to 'inoculation theory,') is hence considered more appropriate towards the goal of prevention.[7] The patient should be encouraged to consider how these images have been doctored, removed from their true context, and designed/presented to encourage consumer dissatisfaction for monetary and/or other gain.

For diabetic patients, another tactic towards evading eating disorders is mollification of the factors that are theorized to contribute towards the pathology. Many of these are marginally iatrogenic in etiology, namely the sometimes overzealous focus on maintaining the HbA1c and blood sugar readings within inflexible and sometimes unattainable margins, encouraging ever more frequent glucose testing, delineating certain 'permissible' and 'unhealthy' foods, promoting weight loss, and lionizing exercise as the diabetes panacea. Most of these, if not all, are considered salient risk factors for development of eating disorders. If not propagated by the treating healthcare professional, this rigid mentality is then likely to be adopted by controlling parents (for younger patients) or the perfectionist patient themselves. Modifying these stringent expectations on all fronts (physician, patient, and/or parents) will aid in attrition of these risk factors, leaving the patient with less predilection towards depression and anxiety. This rigor is especially relevant with regards to glucose control – studies have shown that in an attempt to further decrease HbA1c levels, patients place themselves in greater peril of hypoglycemia. As described, this is a powerful nidus of disordered eating: sourcing binge episodes, apprehension of recurrence, and deliberate underdosing to thwart further hypoglycemia.

Fixating on numbers is also toxic to the psyche – while necessary for the clinician himself to monitor response to therapy, it is perhaps wise to avoid referencing them too frequently during clinic appointments. When the patient is provided a self-calibrated, palpable numerical outcome (such as weight or HbA1c) to trend and fixate upon, they will most likely do so without bidding. Hence (within clinical judgment), the upper limits of 'vague' are preferable to the lower limits of 'specific.' This applies to values considered both within and outside therapeutic goal. Commending the patient – beyond what is considered encouragement for maintenance – for attaining an ideal value only predisposes towards depression if that 'trophy' is breached.

The above concept might be completely inimical to the very tenets of diabetes management (which endorses tight metabolic control to avoid microvascular complications), especially for the parents of young diabetics who feel profoundly responsible not only for their child's current but also future health. Why condone suboptimal (i.e., more lenient) therapy when there is no tenable indication of an eating disorder? *Why coddle the child now when what we should be teaching them is diabetes skills for later years when we won't be there to take care of them? Why sacrifice the concrete for what is not palpable?* Difficult, but legitimate protests for concerned guardians – ultimately, this strategy depends on and must be calibrated according to familial comfort, and will be completely counterproductive if that ideal is compromised.

129

References:

1.) Markowitz, J. T., D. A. Butler, L. K. Volkening, J. E. Antisdel, B. J. Anderson, and L. M.B. Laffel. "Brief Screening Tool for Disordered Eating in Diabetes: Internal Consistency and External Validity in a Contemporary Sample of Pediatric Patients with Type 1 Diabetes." *Diabetes Care* 33.3 (2010): 495-500.

2.) Fairburn, CG; Cooper, Z; Doll, HA; Davies, BA (2005). "Identifying Dieters Who Will Develop an Eating Disorder: A Prospective, Population-Based Study." *The American Journal of Psychiatry* 162 (12): 2249–55.

3.) Eckert, K., Graybar, S. (January 19, 2011). "The treacherous trip from diabetes to eating disorder." Presented at Stanford University Medical Center, Stanford, CA.

4.) D'Emden, Helen, Libby Holden, Brett McDermott, Mark Harris, Anne Gledhill, and Andrew Cotterill. "Concurrent Validity of Self-report Measures of Eating Disorders in Adolescents with Type 1 Diabetes." N.p., n.d. Web.

5.) Wilksch, Simon, Karina Starkey, Anne Gannoni, Tania Kelly, and Tracey Wade. "Interactive Programme to Enhance Protective Factors for Eating Disorders in Girls with Type 1 Diabetes." *Early Intervention in Psychiatry* (2013): 1-7. Web.

6.) O'dea, J., and S. Abraham. "Improving the Body Image, Eating Attitudes, and Behaviors of Young Male and Female Adolescents: A New Educational Approach That Focuses on Self-Esteem." *International Journal of Eating Disorders* 28.1 (2000): 43-57. Print.

7.) Wilksch, Simon M., Mitchell R. Durbridge, and Tracey D. Wade. "A Preliminary Controlled Comparison of Programs Designed to Reduce Risk of Eating Disorders Targeting Perfectionism and Media Literacy." *Journal of the American Academy of Child & Adolescent Psychiatry* 47.8 (2008): 93

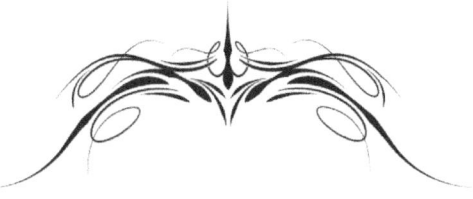

Part III

TOWARDS
HEALING

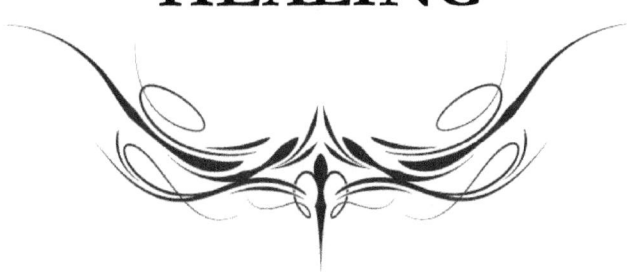

CHAPTER 7

SEQUELAE

There is a certain dangerous arrogance inherent to diabulimia. I always think I know what to expect day after day living with no insulin. Peeing constantly, insatiable thirst, occasional nausea, the air hunger. Every day I survive with only these minor symptoms, my confidence grows, I sail through life because I can eat whatever I want and still stay skinny. The original dread of the cartoon anvil quietly fades, and I actually start to believe that I can perpetuate this.

*One evening I go to pee, and find that there is a pool of froth in the toilet bowl…*No matter, somebody probably just cleaned the bathroom and left some detergent residue in there… *but froth comes the next time, and the next. I am terribly alarmed, and immediately reconnect my insulin pump.* Oh God oh God, what have I done to my kidneys? *But a few days later, the pump lies in the bottom of my sock drawer, spurned into suspension.*

Another day I wake up and put on my slippers before heading to the bathroom, and feel a strange tingling in the tips of my toes that spreads insidiously to the periphery of my feet. The tips of my index fingers and thumbs are slightly numb as well. Maybe I just slept in an odd position. It'll be gone before I take a shower. *It was not. I explain these sensations away, circumvent, rationalize. All the king's horses and all the king's men* could *put Humpty back together again…*

I brush my hair every morning, willing each strand to claw at my scalp for dear life. But they are weak, brittle, and relinquish their hold with nary a battle cry. I can pull them out in tufts, and my once thick mane fades slowly into an anemic pillow of black moss.

But nothing gelled, nothing did enough damage for me to recant, despite the insidious death knells tolling in my wake. I was the overseer, the one in control, the eminence grise. My body was not, and woe to her for attempting to usurp my command. Let her throw at me what she will, but I will thrash her into obedience. She has not given me what I want.

133

The physical complications resulting from diabulimia are not dissimilar to those produced by chronic hyperglycemia, but the concomitant psychological and nutritional detriments of the eating disorder must be considered in tandem. Such additional contributions lend the long-term consequences of this illness much more serious than the sum of these individual elements. Of course, there are a multitude of references available which enumerate the major and minor sequelae of diabetes, but here we discuss them as they pertain specially to diabulimia. Note that these statements, unless specified, are conjectural/theoretical and based on principles of medical pathophysiology. They are yet to be validated in longitudinal clinical trials.

This chapter is partitioned into the three following sections, in reference to effect:

1.) Somatic
2.) Psychiatric
3.) Nutritional

Currently, we can only hypothesize the differences in mortality and morbidity between "restrictive" and "bingeing" diabulimia as described in previous chapters, and posit some qualitative differences in the severity of complications between patterns of omission (e.g. duration, frequency, amplitude). In a 4-5 year follow-up study performed by Rydall et al. (1997), patients were segregated into three groups based on the particular frequency of the following disordered eating patterns: binge eating, insulin manipulation to promote weight loss, self-induced vomiting, or laxative use. The groups were labeled as "highly disordered eating," "moderately disordered eating," and "non-disordered eating." The severity of the complications experienced by each of these populations as well as their glycemic control (as measured by the HbA1c) correlated directly with the extent of their categorized disordered eating.

Extrapolated from this finding is the conjecture that bingeing diabulimia presents a greater risk to the PWDb than purely restrictive diabulimia. Caloric overconsumption places inordinate stress upon the body – not only mechanically but also metabolically. This higher caloric intake in the absence/inadequacy of insulin increases to a greater extent 1.) blood glucose and ketone levels, 2.) kidney exertion, 3.) glycosylation of amino acids and hemoglobin and 4.) toxic accumulation of metabolites such as sorbitol.

Restrictive diabulimia, however, while yet placing stress on all of these systems by virtue of inducing hyperglycemia, glycosuria, and ketonemia/uria, does so to a lesser extent by virtue of decreased caloric intake. Some patients consume so little that even intentionally omitting insulin has a negligible effect because there is minimal substrate in the bloodstream in the first place. 'Restriction,' as such, exerts a relatively more favorable (that is to say, less destructive) influence over the mechanisms contributing to diabetic complications, albeit in dangerous exchange for severe nutritional detriment. That these patients (apart from having severely low BMIs, impaired psychosocial functioning, etc.) might otherwise appear to be completely nondescript in their diabetes management is completely plausible.

Somatic Effects

Type I diabetes infiltrates – to various degrees – almost every aspect of a patient's life. For the conscientious individual, diabetes is a perpetual concern and demands a certain amount of attention. Many people, fortunately, have successfully adapted their lifestyles and attitudes to incorporate these requirements in an appropriate fashion. Others have not been quite as triumphant, and equanimity is relinquished to factors oftentimes beyond the patients' power. It is these individuals from whom a majority of the data on long-term consequences of hyperglycemia are generated. Regarding this population, "hyperglycemia" and "poorly controlled diabetes" are considered synonymous, which is actually misconceived. "Poorly controlled diabetes" implies either 1.) at least some effort towards management, or 2.) predetermination/contemplation, in which the patient acknowledges that they should manage their diabetes better, but such knowledge does not manifest in physical action. It certainly does not entail an *intention* to maintain a hyperglycemic status (as is the situation in diabulimia). For this reason, we cannot infer that because both diabulimia and "poorly controlled diabetes" result in chronic hyperglycemia, the long-term consequences manifest in the two populations will be the same. The metabolic control – and the complications therein – of patients who intentionally induce glycosuria through insulin restriction is theoretically worse than that of any other diabetic subject who suffers from constant hyperglycemia (through unintentional neglect or otherwise). Here, we present data from clinical research literature, and also draw conclusions from unpublished field investigations (e.g. testimonies from real-time patients with diabulimia) so as to illustrate specifically the long-term consequences of this illness.

There are a few studies in the literature which have analyzed the longitudinal clinical outcomes of diabetic patients with eating disorders, and none of them have positive information to relay. The strikingly debilitating consequences of uncontrolled blood sugars – mortality not an insignificant contender – make diabulimia one of the direst combinations of pathologies in existence. High levels of glucose are extremely harmful to almost any physiological system, and we can examine its effects by individual organs. Indeed, finding one that remains unsullied is a singular challenge.

Microvascular damage

The vascular system is transcendent; as such we address it first. In fact, many of the sequelae of what is now labeled diabulimia/ED-DMT1 are categorized in the literature as "microvascular damage," or microangiopathy. This denotes the cumulative injury inflicted on the small blood vessels such as capillaries and vasa vasorum supplying a variety of organs and structures. The reigning mechanism involves irreversible nonenzymatic generation of advanced-glycosylation end products (AGEs), which is a prolonged result of elevated concentrations of glucose in the plasma. (These follow from chain reactions of glucose with free amino acids in circulation or in tissue proteins – similar to the glycation reaction quantified by the HbA1c). AGEs have deleterious effects on 1.) extracellular matrix proteins and 2.) circulating plasma proteins. Formation of AGEs in the extracellular matrix ultimately leads to increased glycoprotein deposition which continues to crosslink with collagen and thicken the vessels' basement membranes, rendering them weak and atypically permeable. AGE-receptor ligation initiates a series of inflammatory cascades which further exacerbate the pathological endothelial porosity, hyaline arteriolosclerosis, and extracellular matrix proliferation.[20] Impaired function of the vessel ensues, posing a significant risk to the organ or nerve it supplies. This status, termed "microangiopathy," is the primary overall source of morbidity that diabulimia entails. Retinopathy, nephropathy, and neuropathy, all of which are detailed below, can each be attributed in part to this general disturbance.

- *Retinopathy*

The eyes in particular are highly vulnerable to destruction in patients with diabulimia for two main reasons: the cells of the retina 1.) unlike other bodily cells (with the exception of neural, kidney, and liver tissue) do not need insulin for glucose entry [6] 2.) are exquisitely vascularized. The clinical glycemic demarcations (e.g. fasting plasma glucose greater than 125 mg/dl, etc.) for diagnosing diabetes are in fact based upon the point at which the risk of developing retinopathy is differentially increased. When the blood sugar is chronically elevated, sorbitol (an end product of excess glucose metabolism in the eye) builds up within the retinal cells. Sorbitol leads to osmotic damage by drawing excess water into the pericytes and causing microaneurysms of retinal vessel endothelium. AGEs likewise accrue in the extracellular fluid, causing the basement membrane of retinal vessels to become thick and functionally impaired.[7] The extensive vascularization of the eye unfortunately makes it relatively more susceptible to microvascular damage from glycosylation products, and in combination with sorbitol accumulation leaves the eye an open target for significant incapacitation. (Other hemodynamic, biochemical, and hormonal abnormalities contribute, but those discussed are the most significant.) This hyperglycemia-induced retinopathy is usually categorized into 1.) non-proliferative (a.k.a. 'background,' also known as 'preproliferative') and 2.) proliferative.

Of the two types, proliferative retinopathy is more advanced and defined clinically by retinal neovascularization. Cell death in the retina secondary to hyperglycemic affront induces a cycle of ischemia and regrowth, ultimately leading to abnormal branching of new blood vessels from existing retinal vascular structures. Although intended as a protective mechanism, formation of these delicate new vessels is eventually followed by their occlusion, rupture, and consequent epithelial proliferation. These preliminary mechanisms in turn spell hemorrhage, macular edema, and retinal detachment/thickening – the overt manifestation of which is visual abnormality and blindness.

Both preproliferative and proliferative diabetic retinopathies are amenable to treatment, which can also prevent the former from progressing to the advanced latter. These treatments primarily include, for prophylaxis as well as cessation of progression, glycemic and blood pressure control (as do most of the standard diabetic complications).[10] Advanced treatment includes surgery for vessel coagulation/cauterization.

A few cohort investigations provide data concerning the prevalence of retinopathy among patients with ED-DMT1, some of whom admitted to using insulin as a purging method. Of the patients who developed microvascular complications in Peveler's study of 87 Type I diabetic patients (2005), 21% had a probable clinical eating disorder, 47% had a history of disordered eating behavior, and 48% had a history of insulin misuse.[9] In Rydall's study of 91 Type I diabetic females (1997), a 4-5 year follow-up revealed that 86% of 'highly' disturbed eaters and 43% of 'moderately' disturbed eaters developed diabetic retinopathy, as compared with 24% of non-disordered eaters.[8]

- *Nephropathy*

The renal system is vastly insulted by the practice of insulin omission. One of the molecular foundations of diabulimia – inducing glycosuria – depends heavily on manipulating the physiological function of the kidney. (Refer to Chapter 3: "Pathophysiology") Without the precise filtrative, reabsorptive, and secretive properties of glomeruli and corticomedullary tubules, diabulimia theoretically would not be viable (or at least largely ineffective). Given its role as cornerstone, the renal system endures significant abuse and potentially permanent damage during the course – and as a result – of the illness.

As with the retina, "microvascular" complications are implicated in the pathogenesis of kidney damage, involving advanced-glycosylation end products that aggregate in renal tissue compartments promoting progressive structural injury. The glomerulus is extensively involved in the hyperglycemic insult to this organ. Secondary to autonomic dysregulation of renal blood pressure and selective hyalinosis of the efferent arteriole, the glomeruli are subject to a debilitating level of exertion. The glomerular filtration rate (GFR) of patients with uncontrolled glucose levels is 25-50% above normal, and the severity of the consequent pathology is roughly proportional to the degree of this hyperfiltration.[11] (It is hypothesized that bingeing diabulimia is more dangerous than restrictive diabulimia when examined from a renal perspective. The greater degree of hyperglycemia in a bingeing PWDb as compared to a restricting PWDb putatively accelerates the glycosylative damage to the glomerulus and microvasculature, thereby more severely compromising overall renal function.) Consequent to the elevated GFR, the glomeruli undergo multiple histological transformations which reduce their ability to function at optimal capacity. The most significant changes are glomerular basement membrane thickening and glomerular hypertrophy/sclerosis. Of these, glomerulosclerosis is considered most influential in destructive capacity, as it culminates in a multitude of kidney-related pathologies, not the least of which is renal failure.[12]

One of the nonspecific indications of glomerular sclerosis is the presence of protein – albumin or creatinine – in the urine. Normally, the walls of the porous glomeruli are lined with anionic glycoproteins which electrochemically inhibit the filtration of the negatively charged plasma proteins. When the glomeruli are damaged due to the pathogenic mechanisms described above, this barrier is disrupted, and large protein molecules are allowed to leak into the filtrate. The presence of albumin in the urine ("albuminuria") is classified as "micro" versus "macro" based on certain concentrations in single samples, or 24-hour urine collection specimens. (The standard of care has currently adopted the protein/creatinine ratio as an acceptable substitute for the 24-hour urine collection for determining existence of pathology.)

The PWDb must realize that aggressive treatment involving insulin therapy and sustained normalization of glucose levels has demonstrated significant benefit for the kidneys. Although not definitive, evidence shows spontaneous regression of *micro*albuminuria to normoalbuminuria following intensive remediation. *Macro*albuminuria, on the other hand, indicates such extensive destruction that spontaneous regression is impossible under any circumstances. During contact with the PWDb already manifesting microalbuminuria (which is actually a significant proportion), clinicians might tactfully emphasize the likelihood that they will progress to irreversible macroalbuminuria and end-stage renal disease if they perpetuate insulin omission. At such a landmark, the only way to avoid accumulation of lethal metabolites, encephalopathy, and death, is commencement of dialysis and/or kidney transplantation.[13]

The literature predicts grave renal consequences of ED-DMT1. For example, in Rydall's 4-5yr follow-up (1997), 43% of diabetic patients with highly disordered eating and 20% with moderately disturbed eating had developed abnormal urinary albumin excretion, as compared with 20% of non-disordered eaters.[8]

- *Neuropathy*

The body's microvasculature also supplies the nervous tissues (mainly the vasa vasorum in the media adventitia, which is the outermost layer of large arteries and veins). Analogous to the eyes and kidneys, damage to this system significantly unhinges neural circuitry. In fact, the same mechanisms implicated in the destruction of the previously described tissues (AGEs and accumulation of sorbitol), are all involved in neuropathic damage secondary to hyperglycemia. Sorbitol causes osmotic damage, inducing demyelination of the Schwann cells supporting peripheral nerves; AGEs likewise damage supplying microvasculature. There are three basic types of neuropathies relevant to diabetes: sensorimotor, autonomic, and mononeuropathy. The longer the net chronicity of hyperglycemia (diabulimia-induced, poorly controlled diabetes, or otherwise), the greater the chance of developing any of the above.

Sensorimotor polyneuropathy is virtually synonymous with the vernacular "diabetic neuropathy." It is the most prevalent type of neuropathy in this demographic; vice versa, diabetic individuals also constitute the greatest percentage of patients with the condition. Gradual destruction of neuronal axons translates to loss of sensation, tingling, numbness, 'burning' pain, as well as involuntary muscle twitching (fasciculations) primarily in the distal feet and legs.

Autonomic neuropathy is also widespread among patients with diabetes, and engenders an array of secondary pathologies. This condition affects virtually any and all organ systems innervated by the autonomic nervous system, inducing derangements which usually are asymptomatic until advanced. A startling number of diabulimia patients – advanced or otherwise – suffer an array of impairments. Cardiovascular abnormalities include tachycardia (fast heart rate due to impaired parasympathetic discharge) and orthostatic hypotension (dizziness upon standing due to impaired sympathetic discharge). Effects on the gastrointestinal tract include gastroparesis (delayed gastric emptying due to vagal nerve damage, which causes nausea and vomiting), gastroesophageal reflux disease (impaired innervation of the esophageal sphincters), and chronic diarrhea/constipation (gastrointestinal hypomotility secondary to damaged nerves in the abdominal plexus). Genitourinary nerve damage most commonly manifests as bladder voiding/retention problems, and sexual impotence. One particularly important consequence of autonomic neuropathy is the failure to recognize low blood sugars. The somatic symptoms of hypoglycemia (such as tachycardia, sweating, and tremor) are mediated by both parasympathetic and sympathetic divisions of the autonomic nervous system. Without functional innervation, these warning signs are obtunded and hypoglycemia might not be addressed until too late.[22] Gangrene is a delayed chronological sequelae of autonomic neuropathy, but not an uncommon one – diffuse damage of nerves and blood vessels in extremities causes necrosis and dysfunction of the dependent tissues, sometimes requiring amputation.

'Mononeuropathy' is damage to a single nerve. In diabetes/diabulimia the most commonly affected are those supplying the extraocular muscles, namely cranial nerves III (oculomotor), IV (trochlear) and VI (abducens). Compromise manifests as double vision and/or drooping of the eyelids.

Fortunately, neuropathy is not a self-propagating condition (unlike macroalbuminuria and other diabetes-induced renal complications), and once manifest can still be halted or even spontaneously reversed (although the latter is less common). The main factor implicated in these beneficial effects is aggressive glycemic normalization and sustained control; other treatments have not yet been validated.[14] Unfortunately, there is no specific

141

data in the literature to validate the course of neuropathies in diabulimia patients, but anecdotally most have been observed. Gastroparesis (autonomic) is very common, as is sensorimotor neuropathy, orthostatic hypotension, and hypoglycemic oblivion. Mononeuropathy is documented, but not to the degree of severity or frequency as the other subtypes.

- *Lipid Abnormalities*

Dyslipidemia is prematurely accelerated in patients with Type I diabetes. Investigators in one study demonstrated that increasing blood glucose levels were in direct proportion to fasting plasma lipid levels (cholesterol, triglycerides, low-density lipoproteins (LDLs), and very-low-density-lipoproteins (VLDLs).[2] Likewise, another study showed that elevated HbA1c levels likewise correlated directly with increases in VLDL, LDL, and triglycerides, while concomitantly reducing the amount of HDL (considered the 'beneficial cholesterol').[3]

A few studies have also shown that the blood lipid levels of newly diagnosed children/adolescents are markedly elevated.[23] This finding is of specific interest here, as the PWDb mimics this pre-diagnosis period in order to lose or control weight. This state entails 1.) absence of insulin, and 2.) excessive hyperglycemia. Both are implicated in the aforementioned findings for this newly diagnosed population, and, likewise, the PWDb. The absence of insulin inhibits the utilization of glucose, which forces the body to cannibalize its reservoir of adipose tissue to effect energy production. This generates an anomalous accumulation of lipid metabolites in the blood, such as LDLs, VLDLs, cholesterols, and triglycerides. Insulin also plays a role in activating the lipoprotein lipase enzyme which hydrolyzes triglycerides, thereby promoting their cellular uptake and ultimately decreasing the plasma triglyceride levels. Insulin deficiency in diabulimia precludes this normal physiological process and stimulates hypertriglyceridemia (which in newly diagnosed patients is generally reversible upon institution of insulin therapy).

Although, to our knowledge, there are no studies examining dyslipidemias in diabetic patients with eating disorders, interviews with individuals suffering from diabulimia have testified to its presence. Patients in remission/recovery have reported that a few years or even months adhering to a healthy diet and suitable insulin/glucose control have rectified any abnormalities in lipid levels.

- ***Diabetic Ketoacidosis (DKA)***

The pathophysiology of this condition is discussed in Chapter 4. Cerebral edema and coma are two major outcomes of DKA, and in some situations might prove fatal. Cerebral edema typically occurs only in the pediatric demographic, but is still an outcome in older adolescent (diabulimia demographic) patients. Coma is rare, but imminent if treatment is extensively delayed – signs such as Kussmaul breathing and stupor/obtundation should necessitate immediate evaluation. In most cases, however, DKA is resolved sans long-term complications (sequelae from chronic hyperglycemia notwithstanding).

We must emphasize that no physiological system is immune from the deadly effects of hyperglycemia and insulin absence induced by diabulimia. The skin, liver, heart, brain – all are susceptible to hyperglycemic insult and pose crippling risks to the PWDb. These complications might result from mechanisms similar to those described for the more well-documented outcomes, as well as by biodynamics specific to the organ itself.

On the whole, the prospect for improving/reversing these sequelae (minus proliferative retinopathy and macroalbuminuria) with insulin therapy should be gradually underscored to the PWDb if they or their physicians seek further impetus to commence treatment. These outcomes are evident on a spectrum for each patient – those more fortunate might suffer from mild tingling in the fingertips or transiently blurry vision, but for others the symptoms can be expressly frightening and in some cases incapacitating. Although it is generally counterproductive to threaten a further deterioration with perpetuation of adverse behaviors, outlining the possibility for stasis or improvement certainly is not.

Psychiatric Effects

Apart from somatic complications, diabulimia also has documented psychiatric effects, present both during and after extended remission. Various studies have demonstrated that Type I diabetes (without eating disorders/insulin omission) leads to clinical depression, in as much as 30% of the populations under scrutiny.[15,16] Anecdotally, depression can be present during the course of diabulimia as well as the period closely following recovery, but attenuates following extended periods of proper insulin therapy. Distinguishing causality is important here: depression might induce sub-optimal glycemic management, but poor glucose control is likewise capable of provoking depression through physiological effects of hyperglycemia on the brain and psyche.

The presence of an eating disorder – insulin-restricting or otherwise – only exacerbates the incidence of other psychiatric disorders. Pollock et al. (1995) determined that eating-disordered Type I diabetic patients (4% of which demonstrated diabulimia symptoms at baseline) were nine times more likely to suffer or have suffered from a psychiatric disorder such as depression, anxiety, and substance abuse during the 9-year follow-up interval.[18] An 11-year follow-up study of originally insulin-restricting patients performed recently by Goebel-Fabbri et al. (2011), reveals an encouraging result in that patients who ceased omitting insulin demonstrated lower levels of both diabetes-specific as well as overall psychological distress.[19]

Psychological repercussions pertaining to metabolic control in the post-recovery period are also important to consider. Oftentimes, diabulimia patients with chronic insulin misuse will have developed some of the classic diabetes-induced pathologies mentioned above, however prematurely. The presence of these complications, as well as the added frustration of dealing with diabetes management again (which might be highly refractory after extended periods of time without insulin) provide little to no validation of the worth of perseverance. Adverse physical changes manifesting post-treatment, such as weight gain and edema, aggravate circumstances even further. The holistic situation in some cases leads to dangerous suicidal ideations.

Cyclical weight gain is another detrimental consequence of diabulimia resulting in long-term psychological ramifications. Etiologies of increased body mass include a) binge episodes, which might not be completely negated by the insulin restriction pattern of choice, b) phases of remission and relapse, resulting in residual edema from each progressive cycle, c) caloric restriction patterns which might trigger overeating in a period of insulin normality ('abstinence-violation' principle). In an eating disorder category generally populated by patients of ostensibly normal BMI (in contrast to the prototypically perceived 'underweight eating-disordered' patient), the upward-trending vacillation in mass even renders patients overweight. This potentially exacerbates disturbed eating behaviors as well as the impetus to insulin manipulation, leading to severe incapacitation and/or mortality. In Goebel-Fabbri et al.'s 11-year follow-up study (2011) of originally insulin-restricting patients, women who reported continued insulin restriction demonstrated increased BMI levels. Ironically (and perhaps counterintuitively), women who ceased insulin manipulation actually had stable BMI's at the follow-up period.[19]

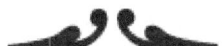

Nutritional Consequences

The nutritional sequelae of diabulimia do not exactly mimic those of standard eating disorders such as purely non-insulin-omitting anorexia and diabulimia nervosas. They certainly do overlap unidirectionally, in that eating-disordered insulin-omitting patients will generally suffer the complications of malnourishment as well as complications of uncontrolled diabetes.

Whether or not the PWDb is categorized as restrictive or bingeing, they are essentially in a profound state of starvation. Similar to the pre-diagnosis period, insulin absence precludes physical nourishment despite excessive caloric intake. Through purging with insulin omission, diabulimia patients self-induce conditions of malnourishment even in the absence of other compensatory methods. The major complications affecting non-diabetic eating-disordered patients collateral to dietary restriction are therefore fair game for any PWDb. These include, most commonly, menstrual irregularities, osteoporosis, and dental deterioration. Others are cerebral atrophy, immunocompromise, cardiac malady, and dermatological abnormalities.

Electrolyte imbalances especially are acutely exacerbated in the absence of insulin (vomiting, laxative/diuretic use notwithstanding). Hyperglycemia induces an osmotic diuresis by creating a hyperosmolar glomerular filtrate, which decreases reabsorption of water in the renal tubules (functioning exactly like a pharmacological osmotic diuretic such as mannitol). Inhibition of water reabsorption concomitantly results in the excretion of other important molecules (such as potassium, calcium, magnesium, phosphate, chloride, and others). In general, the polyuria induced by both hyperglycemia and/or the pathological use of diuretics overrides the fine-tuned dynamics that the body has instituted to maintain serum electrolytes, culminating in inappropriate retention *and* elimination of particular substances. As myriad physiological processes depend on proper serum concentrations of these ions, imbalances are rapidly toxic.

The modus operandi of insulin omission might stratify the severity of these complications depending on whether it permits the body to metabolize an adequate amount of calories. For example, a patient who only omits their insulin for one meal would not be purging the rough entirety of their other meals. Although the same principle does not apply to electrolytes, vitamins, or other micronutrients due to their sensitivity to renal elimination mechanisms, it is generally applicable towards macronutrients such as carbohydrates, fat, and proteins, the breakdown of which is inhibited by the presence of insulin (to certain extents, depending on the serum concentration of the hormone).

Diabulimia need not present with a clinically low BMI, and very often actually does not. Nevertheless, this is always a possibility. There are two qualifications between patient groups to be made here: those who 1.) *present* at any time with low BMI, which consists of both restricting and bingeing PWDbs, and 2.) *develop* a low BMI, which is more often than not only the restrictive PWDbs. The distinction here is made upon the basis of *change* in weight. This is to say that both restrictive and bingeing patients can "commence" diabulimia with dangerously low BMIs. However, it is difficult for a bingeing PWDb to lose weight longitudinally, given the nature of bingeing practices. On the other hand, restrictive PWDbs, who excessively curtail caloric intake, *as well as* purge with insulin omission, can *develop* dangerously low body weight. (These patients represent the minority of PWDbs, however.) This derives from a qualitative difference between bingeing and restriction in the body's activation of emergency survival systems. In a bingeing PWDb, energy production can source from the marginal amount of calories that the body absorbs during the caloric excess of binge excursions (although the vast majority still spills into the urine) despite hypoinsulinemia; their endogenous tissues are relatively spared until advanced stages. In a restrictive PWDb, this alternate supply of ingested calories is nigh eliminated, and in the absence of insulin the body resorts to dismantling of fat and muscle, leading to compounded weight loss. Amenorrhea, low bone density, hormonal/neurological/cardiovascular abnormalities, infertility, and anemia can all ensue, dampening both the medical prognosis as well as patient quality of life.

References:
1.) Chance GW, Albutt EC, Edkins SM: Serum lipids and lipoproteins in untreated diabetic children. *Lancet* 1:1126–1128, 1969
2.) Sosenko JM, Breslow JL, Miettinen OS, Gabbay KH: Hyperglycemia and plasma lipid levels, a prospective study of young insulin-dependent diabetic patients. *New England Journal of Medicine* 302:650–654, 1980
3.) Lopes-Virella MF, Wohltmann HJ, Loadholt CB, Buse MG: Plasma lipids and lipoproteins in young insulin-dependent diabetic patients: relationship with control. *Diabetologia* 21:216–223, 1981
4.) Wiltshire, E. J., C. Hirte, and J. J. Couper. "Dietary Fats Do Not Contribute to Hyperlipidemia in Children and Adolescents With Type 1 Diabetes." *Diabetes Care* 26 (2003): 1356-361.
5.) Chait, Alan, and Karin Bornfeldt. "Diabetes and Atherosclerosis: Is There a Role for Hyperglycemia?" Journal of Lipid Research, Supplement (2009): S335-339. Web.
6.) Lansel, N., and G. Niemeyer. "Effects of Insulin Under Normal and Low Glucose on Retinal Electrophysiology in the Perfused Cat Eye." *Investigative Ophthalmology & Visual Science* 38.5 (1997).
7.) McCullogh, D. "Pathogenesis of Diabetic Retinopathy." *UptoDate*. 29 Apr. 2009
8.) Rydall A, Rodin G, Olmsted M, Devenyi R, Daneman D. Disordered Eating Behavior and Microvascular Complications in Young Women with Insulin-Dependent Diabetes Mellitus. *New England Journal of Medicine* 1997; 336: 1849-854.

9.) Peveler, R. C., K. S. Bryden, H. A. W. Neil, C. G. Fairburn, R. A. Mayou, D. B. Dunger, and H. M. Turner. "The Relationship of Disordered Eating Habits and Attitudes to Clinical Outcomes in Young Adult Females With Type 1 Diabetes." *Diabetes Care*28.1 (2005): 84-88.

10.) "Progression of Retinopathy with Intensive versus Conventional Treatment in the Diabetes Control and Complications Trial. Diabetes Control and Complications Trial Research Group." *Ophthalmology* 102 (1995): 647-61.

11.) Bank, Norman. "Mechanisms of Diabetic Hyperfiltration." *Kidney International* 40.4 (1991): 792-807.

12.) Tuttle KR, Bruton JL, Perusek MC, Lancaster JL, Kopp DT, DeFronzo RA. "Effect of Strict Glycemic Control on Renal Hemodynamic Response to Amino Acids and Renal Enlargement in Insulin-dependent Diabetes Mellitus." *New England Journal of Medicine* 324.23 (1991): 1626.

13.) McCullogh, D., and G. Bakris. "Microalbuminuria." *UptoDate.* 10 Aug. 2010.

14.) Feldman, E. L. "Epidemiology and Classification of Diabetic Neuropathy." *UptoDate.* 12 Aug. 2009.

15.) Stewart S, Rao U, Emslie G, Klein D, White P. Depressive Symptoms Predict Hospitalization for Adolescents with Type I Diabetes. Pediatrics 2005; 115: 1315-319.

16.) Zhang X, Norris S, Gregg E, Cheng Y, Beckles G, Khan H. Depressive Symptoms and Mortality among Persons with and without Diabetes. *American Journal of Epidemiology* 2005; 161: 652-50.

17.) Musselman D, Betan E, Larsen H, Phillips L. Relationship of Depression to Diabetes Types I and 2: Epidemiology, Biology, and Treatment. *Biological Psychiatry* 2003; 54: 317-29.

18.) Pollock, Myrna, Maria Kovacs, and Denise Charron-Prochownik. "Eating Disorders and Maladaptive Dietary/Insulin Management among Youths with Childhood-Onset Insulin-Dependent Diabetes Mellitus." *Journal of the American Academy of Child & Adolescent Psychiatry* 34.3 (1995): 291.

19.) Goebel-Fabbri, A., B. Anderson, D. Franko, J. Fikkan, K. Pearson, and K. Weinger. "Improvement and Emergence of Insulin Restriction in Women With Type 1 Diabetes."*Diabetes Care* 34 (2011): 545-50.

20.) Robbins, Stanley L., Vinay Kumar, and Ramzi S. Cotran. *Robbins and Cotran Pathologic Basis of Disease.* Philadelphia, PA: Saunders/Elsevier, 2010. Print.

21.) "Hyperglycemia: a Risk Factor in Coronary Heart Disease." *Circulation* 36 (1967): 609-19.

22.) Vinik, A. I., R. E. Maser, B. D. Mitchell, and R. Freeman. "Diabetic Autonomic Neuropathy."*Diabetes Care* 26.5 (2003): 1553-579.

23.) Chase, PH, and AM Glasgow. "Juvenile Diabetes Mellitus and Serum Lipids and Lipoprotein Levels." *Am J Dis Child* 10 (1979): 1113-117. Print.

24.) Nikkila, EA, and P. Hormila. "Serum Lipids and Lipoproteins in Insulin-treated Diabetes."*Diabetes* 27 (1978): 1078-086. Web.

CHAPTER 8

TREATMENT

*Have you ever seen an advertisement for one of those Tempur-pedic "memory"
mattresses? Where you press down on the ergonomically designed material with your
palm, and it stays depressed in that shape for a good 6 or 7 seconds before rising up
again? It's like that. It's almost terrifying, how Tempur-pedic our extremities, our
forearms, legs, ankles, fingers, face can become. The doctors call it "pitting edema," but I
always thought that was laughably pompous.*

*The week after going back on insulin is actually the worst. We start out with an
already skewed perception of our bodies, and adding the extra pounds of water to the
weight we believe we have lost is mentally devastating, especially since it appears within
the window of only a few days. It looks heavy, feels even heavier...worst of all it makes us
question seriously our reasons for wanting to take insulin again. We, who feel more
profoundly the aberrant bite of dry cracker and punish ourselves for it, for what will never
even register — where do we cower, where do we shout and retreat when this is thrown
upon us all at once? It is frighteningly easy to look at our suddenly bloated bodies in the
mirror, feel the thickness of our ankles that were so bony and angular just yesterday, and
become so panicked such that the insulin shot is foregone, the blood sugar kit is thrown
under the bed, the pump disconnected.*

*The "pitting edema" eventually fades away, but not fast enough for us to realize it
in any rational capacity. It takes every filament of our being, every hoax we can pull upon
ourselves, everything we have ever lived for and will live for and look forward to... to
wrench ourselves to plunge needle after needle into those bulbous limbs...*

Towards Healing

While suffering from insulin omission and its complications, the PWDb might wish to take manage their diabetes again. Unfortunately, these motivations are significantly encumbered not only by intrinsic mental sabotage but also the adverse physical manifestations of recovery processes. During attempts at self-treatment, they will frequently cycle between intervals (lasting for hours, days, weeks – ad infinitum) of insulin compliance and non-adherence. In the words of one patient: *"Diabulimia has become such an intertwined part of my life – I can't ever really say that I'm in recovery because it's hard to differentiate from total normality. If I'm not acting it out, then it's in my head. Of course, much of the time, it's in my head, and I'm acting it out as well..."* Depending on the patient's psychiatric and pathologic baselines, this interval of compliance is curtailed by isolated cognitions, or those prompted by the materialization of specific physical symptoms (edema, hypoglycemia, weight gain, pain, caloric restriction). As such, treatment is also characterized by deep antagonism towards either the entire concept or just specific nuances of the recovery process.

A desire to improve, no matter how chronically ambivalent, is the first step towards recovery. It is a thoroughly arduous process requiring concentrated dedication from not only the patient but also their clinical and familial/social environments. The conviction that "It's all up to them – if they want to get better then they'll get better" is a hazardously inaccurate assessment, as extrinsic factors are equally important as those intrinsic. However, suffice it to say that if the patient *does not* want to recover, they most definitely will not – no matter the degree of external coaxing or duress. This is one of the problems facing the medical world – what is the purpose of recognition if the patient themselves is not amenable to change? Why must we work towards increasing external awareness if subsequent encouragement towards recovery falls upon deaf ears? Where those aware are now tormented by the knowledge that they are powerless?

Manipulative fright tactics are fundamentally counterproductive. Patients have either developed such profound sentiments of apathy that threatening even the most dire consequences will do little to sway them. Cowing a PWDb with ultimatums like "Do you want to end up blind, in kidney failure, or dead?," "You're never going away to college if you continue like this," or "Do want us to suffer with anxiety over your health?" can lead to further antagonism, not to mention 'defiance' omission to reinforce control. The average adolescent subpopulation generally mentates concretely rather than abstractly, i.e. it is more difficult for them to project penalties of immediate actions; this precludes any traction of threat. In some cases, patients have already developed crippling sequelae, and there is little else that can incite the intended trepidation.

Coercion is likewise a futile principle. If the PWDb is forced into rehabilitation and subsequently 'healed,' the return to an uncontrolled environment will only enable them to resume destructive behaviors. The mind – *not* the body – is the culprit here. Clinicians in the diabetic team must be aware of these complex internal circumstances and apply that awareness to individualized treatment strategies. These are profoundly frustrating circumstances for the physician especially – who many times has no choice but to watch their patient spiral downwards into failing health and deteriorating psychology, helpless to contribute anything other than recommendations or prescriptions. They might progressively enable the patient to adopt a more amenable attitude towards diabulimia therapy, but too often such acquiescence is determined by processes beyond their power.

Managed care organizations are another significant barrier for hospitalization, eating disorder program admission, and outpatient medicine, as they sometimes do not validate the frameworks necessary for successful treatment (including eligibility criteria, multidisciplinary work, extended lengths of inpatient stay, certain medications or treatment modalities), leading to overall mediocre/curtailed therapy. The concept of secondary and tertiary prevention is thus abandoned. This further has ramifications on readmission rates, patient prognosis, and longitudinal healthcare costs (sequelae of diabulimia such as kidney disease, retinopathy, etc., which must then be chronically managed and necessitate even more aggressive treatment). PWDbs themselves, whether they classify as dependents or independents under insurance plans, are fettered by the sometimes staggering monetary stipulations, choosing to forego treatment altogether.

Inpatient Treatment

Diabulimia, once recognized, can be treated in either an inpatient or outpatient setting. There is unfortunately a paucity of studies comparing the value of either method for just anorexia nervosa or bulimia nervosa, let alone a diabetes-specific eating disorder such as diabulimia. (Likewise, there is sparse solid data on the incidence of diabulimia/ED-DMT1 recovery itself – the only information on long- and short-term recuperation is primarily through clinical narrative.) Some physicians believe that an outpatient setting for the purposes of recovery is preferable because it places the patient directly in an antagonistic environment during the course of their rehabilitation. The inpatient milieu, on the other hand, is more secluded and, while enforcing potent medical stabilization, does not successfully expose the patient to the anti-recovery elements present in the public setting. In the case of adolescent patients, it also fails to harness the skills of parents and siblings, who might be trained to help prolong recovery after discharge. The PWDb might also attempt to extend their stay within the inpatient center to avoid returning to the "real world," elements of which perhaps triggered their illness in the first place. A study from Japan did report upon a 3-year follow-up that their particular 'integrated inpatient therapy' involving both psychotherapeutic counseling and medical management for ED-DMT1 patients was associated with reductions in HbA1c levels, depression, anxiety, and behavioral disturbances related to eating disorders (compared to isolated outpatient therapy).[28]

In general, inpatient rehabilitation is reserved for physically or psychiatrically unstable patients, who after discharge are treated with suitable courses of outpatient treatment. This encompasses individuals who are severely underweight, presenting as a danger to themselves or others, or manifesting symptoms of severe dehydration, electrolyte abnormality, or autonomic dysfunction. Treatment for insulin-omitting eating disorders is generally more common in the outpatient setting from the onset (but this observation may be biased due to lack of recognition within inpatient rehabilitation centers). Patients might also themselves elect to join an inpatient eating disorder recovery program. This is complicated by specific facility exclusions, which might stipulate a no-admittance policy for "high-risk" or "constant medical attention-requiring" patients, criteria of which diabulimia patients unfortunately often meet.

DKA is most often the acute presenting pathology, for which there is a specific stabilization protocol. This includes vascular fluid resuscitation with a low-grade insulin infusion, which antagonizes further ketone formation and furthers their urinary elimination. The blood sugar level will usually correct before ketone levels are normalized, necessitating intravenous dextrose supplementation and higher levels of insulin which are necessary to completely eradicate residual ketones and completely close the anion gap they have created. Electrolytes are monitored carefully, as profound dehydration followed by reinstitution of fluid and insulin yields the patient dangerously hypokalemic (which itself can lead to lethal cardiac arrhythmias). Supportive treatment is provided (until ketone levels and arterial blood gases are normalized), urine output measured to monitor kidney function, and blood sugars closely observed. (The current criteria for DKA in both the adult and pediatric population includes documentation of hyperglycemia (greater than 200 mg/dl in children, and generally greater than 250 mg/dl in adults). These are PWDbs, who – whether or not they have experienced prior DKA episodes – attempt desperately to compensate by giving themselves rapid and excessive amounts of insulin. This is not an uncommon practice – trying frantically to reverse DKA with insulin is gravely logical but also gravely perilous. This renders them normoglycemic or even *hypo*glycemic. During emergency department triage, this incongruous symptom might dangerously delay or confound treatment.)

One of the problems with DKA as the cause of inpatient admission is the fact that it is usually treated as a garden-variety medical problem, sans accounting for either/both of 1.) malnutrition, or 2.) psychological duress. As such, monitoring frameworks or clinical pathways specific to eating disorders (such as weight gain, caloric scrutiny and compliance, bed rest) is not regularly performed because inpatient clinicians are unaware or seek to discharge the patient as soon as legitimately possible. Perfunctory workups are performed in order to locate a potential precipitant for the ketoacidosis (e.g., gastroenteritis, urinary tract infection, pneumonia, etc.), the absence of which will only falsely reassure the PWDb that their act of omitting insulin was relatively benign. In a medically emergent state such as DKA, further exacerbation secondary to this suboptimal monitoring can prove perilous to the patient, not to mention leading to higher readmission rates and worse long-term prognosis.

While in the hospital for eating disorder/diabulimia treatment, the PWDb's diet is monitored closely as pertaining to weight trajectory, similar to other non-diabetic patients hospitalized for the same reason. They are provided a predetermined daily caloric intake (through nasogastric tube if the patient refuses or cannot tolerate oral intake, as they do if prevented from omitting their insulin) in order to gradually append or maintain stable weight. As a precaution, patients are placed under close surveillance after meals and in the bathroom to prevent further purging behaviors.

Inpatient treatment elicits variable degrees of resistance from the PWDb, and as such, physicians have invented a few methods to neutralize refractory behavior. One major problem is the administration of insulin – as detailed in Chapter 5, the PWDb has an arsenal of deceptive mechanisms designed to eliminate doses. Some bingeing PWDbs, on the other hand, resent the controlled food intake environment, and might subsequently administer themselves excess insulin. This entitles (indeed, almost forces) them to transiently increase intake until their blood sugar is normalized – essentially mimicking a binge. Depending on hospital policy, Type I patients are either allowed to continue using their pumps while within the wards, or use insulin injections with boluses, sliding scales, and long-acting basal insulin as a complete replacement (which allegedly makes for easier medical documentation). As such, patients are sometimes allowed to give themselves their own injections for comfort, which for a PWDb must be avoided. Nurses or certified hospital staff must administer all insulin.

Outpatient Treatment

The outpatient treatment process for an insulin-omitting eating disorder is multidisciplinary, involving generally no less than an endocrinologist, dietician, and mental health professional; sometimes a diabetes educator or registered nurse are included. Ideally, all members (particularly the dietician and/or nurse) will have experience in the treatment of eating disorders, but this is not always feasible. Incorporating expertise from each of these fields is ideal for instituting a viable plan towards long-term recuperation. Often the patient's primary care physician will coordinate the various clinicians comprising the 'diabetic team,' ensuring that they communicate extensively so that each understands the occurrences, implications, and intentions of the other members' clinical assessments and treatments. This synchronism effects productive modifications on all fronts of mental and physical recovery.

For certain reasons, some components of this team are completely absent, or have suboptimal levels of intercommunication. The 'diabetic team' dictum in some circumstances is not yet optimized, or is – wrongly – considered categorically unnecessary. The patient in this case must become their own advocate – documenting recommendations, labs, medications, so as to ensure that everyone is adequately informed. Unfortunately, transmission of information in this manner is not always comprehensively realized, as certain vital values and assessments/plans might fall through the cracks or even be intentionally withheld by the PWDb.

Insulin Therapy

Insulin therapy is the first area to be conquered (chronologically). Although some might argue that psychotherapy is more important given the potent mental provenance of the condition, immediate implementation is futile given the often severe hyperglycemia present before treatment. Patients simply do not have normal cognition at these blood glucose levels, which are often too "HI" (glucose kit-speak for 'high') for the blood glucose meter to even detect. Concentration, reasoning, deductive abilities, even insight (the ability of the patient to recognize their own pathology) – all are variably impaired with gross hyperglycemia. Commencing a course of psychiatric treatment is hence counterproductive unless glucose values are appreciably lowered. Once these decrease to at least a consistent 200-250 mg/dl (anecdotal values), psychotherapy is feasibly initiated based on the team's judgment. During this time, concomitant nutritional restitution will also enhance insight and mentation, better priming the patient.

One of the most important axioms arising from the reinstitution of insulin therapy with a PWDb is that of gradation. It is essential that the blood sugar be decreased in incremental amounts (as opposed to a fell plunge towards euglycemia) for multiple physiological and psychological reasons:

1.) Diabulimia patients have been under hyperglycemic influence for such extended periods that their epistat becomes intimately accustomed to the resulting conditions. Consequently, a normal blood sugar level will induce hypoglycemic symptoms unless the body can acclimatize slowly to a new, non-pathological baseline. For example, 215mg/dl after living chronically in the range of 600-700mg/dl might be perceived as 60 mg/dl - stimulating the cholinergic/adrenergic constellation of tremors, confusion, palpitations, and sweating. Patients who are 'brought down' too quickly also experience depression, nausea, and listlessness (in addition to hypoglycemic symptoms). These effects are attributed both to autonomic nervous system subversion as well as the acutely lower *relative* concentration of glucose supplying the brain (i.e., compared to the prior hyperglycemia).

2.) Insulin is a powerful edematogenic agent, and its administration can result in fluid retention of 5-15 pounds lasting from a few days to a few months. In addition (insulin notwithstanding), patients have been so chronically dehydrated secondary to hyperglycemia and ketoacidosis that even acute treatment for DKA with intravenous fluids can append another 5-10 pounds. This response takes devastating tolls on the already hypersensitive psyche of patients embarking on the long road towards recovery. Giving insulin incrementally over the period of a few weeks/months potentially diminishes the amount of edema or renders it less acute.[10]

---

[10]   **Pathophysiology of insulinogenic edema**

One of the most terrifying aspects of the journey towards recovery from diabulimia (and occasionally non-insulin-omitting eating disorders) is the edema– a diabolical swelling of almost any joint, axial limb, central cavity, and extremity that accompanies reinstitution of insulin therapy and nutritional correction. Fluid accumulates in interstitial bodily cavities and effects a weight gain ranging from 5-15 pounds. This can appear days to weeks after insulin dosing is resumed, and persist for days to months. Considering that the minimal prerequisite for recognition of peripheral edema is an extracellular volume expansion of 2 liters (4.5 pounds), a further *visible* expansion translates to almost an extra 15 pounds of body mass. The edema is generally relative to original body mass such that, *all else equal,* a heavier individual will gain proportionally more absolute mass than a lighter one (such that the final manifestations are similar). This is an extremely distressing cognitive phenomenon for the PWDb, as it is not immediately evident that the water retention is only a temporary compensatory mechanism. They are already extremely sensitive to fluctuations in weight, and the body's post-treatment convention of appending an extra few pounds of painfully perceptible fluid is psychologically paralyzing.

The pathophysiology of this particular type of edema is complex, and it derives from a combination of processes. These are initiated by 1.) introduction of insulin into the system, and/or 2.) the process of lowering the blood glucose and maintaining it at a normal level. Although there is more scientific evidence to support the former, a more viable hypothesis involves their mutual interaction in producing the overall manifestation of edema.

The most highly documented corollary of insulin treatment is retention of sodium, the precise pathogenesis of which remains to be elucidated. Multiple investigations have demonstrated impaired natriuresis following reinstitution of insulin, leading to higher levels of sodium in the extracellular fluid. The general consensus is renal hyperabsorption, but the precise anatomic tubular location is still to be pinpointed.[2] Reservation of this particular electrolyte is accompanied by fluid accumulation in both blood plasma and extracellular fluid. One theory involves the insulin-glucagon-aldosterone relationship. Insulin and glucagon engage in a mutually inhibitory fashion – the presence of insulin dampens the release and action of glucagon, and vice versa. During times of complete or drastically lowered insulin absence, such as 1.) pre-diagnosis, 2.) "poorly controlled diabetes," or 3.) diabulimia, levels of glucagon are elevated. Among other crucial functions, one of the actions of glucagon is to increase natriuresis by inhibiting the effects of circulating aldosterone.[14] (This is one of the explanations for the loss of water during normal fasting – the body signals for the secretion of glucagon so as protect against hypoglycemia secondary to decreased intake; the glucagon induces sodium excretion, followed by water excretion. People undertaking fad 'starvation' diets experience dramatic weight loss during the first few days, which is partially attributed to this biodynamic.) Re-introduction of insulin dampens circulating glucagon, and alleviates the aldosterone inhibition, which ultimately results in sodium retention, plasma expansion, and concomitant edema.[11]

A key point is that this sodium retention phenomenon appears to be dependent on *both* the plasma insulin *as well as blood glucose level*. In a study by Fioretto et al., researchers studied sodium dynamics under three different conditions: 1.) a conventional insulin regimen during which plasma glucose was approximately 210 mg/dl, and plasma insulin 27 µU/ml, 2.) an intensified insulin regimen with strict metabolic control during which plasma glucose was decreased to approximately 115 mg/dl and plasma insulin was increased to approximately 44 µU/ml, and 3.) an intensified insulin regimen similar to #2 where plasma insulin was 48 µU/ml but where the plasma glucose was maintained at an elevated level between 225 and 270 mg/dl. As expected, the excretion of sodium was greater under condition #1. However, it is interesting to note that a comparison between the normoglycemic (#2) and hyperglycemic (#3) but hyperinsulinemic states revealed that the sodium excretion rate was significantly lower for the normoglycemic state. The result implies that an isolated state of normoglycemia even in the absence of hyperinsulinemia itself can effect appreciable sodium retention.[1] This finding is especially germane to the issue of diabulimia recovery, which involves both 1.) administration of exogenous insulin and 2.) induction of normoglycemia (which is partially dependent on exogenous insulin administration). This also has implications for the chronicity and incrementality of diabulimia therapy.

Elevated vasopressin (anti-diuretic hormone) concentrations induced by the chronic hyperglycemic osmotic diuresis cannot downscale at an appreciable rate after normoglycemia is achieved, leading also to inappropriate water retention.[12] It is in the patient's best interest to effect both these endeavors gradually if severely acute sodium retention and concomitant increase in extracellular fluid volume is to be attenuated. For example, a suitable course of action begins with low doses of insulin adequate for slight lowering of the blood glucose level, and gradual increases are implemented over the course of a few days/weeks (depending on the patient's physiological responses) until euglycemia is achieved. If the clinician is concerned about the further perpetuation of hyperglycemia that this method entails, they should consider the much higher likelihood of short/long-term relapse if the PWDb is subject to severe edema.

A concept inherent to the pathogenesis of edema is Starling's equation, which describes the directionality of fluid movement across capillary membranes. It defines the net movement of fluid from the vascular space into the extracellular compartment as a function of the dominance of interstitial hydrostatic forces (fluid movement *out of* the capillary) over capillary oncotic forces (fluid movement from the interstitium *into* the capillary). Both pressures depend on an array of variables, but for edema the relevant parameter is the intravascular albumin concentration, which directly determines the magnitude of the oncotic force. Insulin treatment induces escape of albumin from this compartment, by pathologically increasing vascular permeability.[15,16] The capillary oncotic pressure is thereby reduced and results in an overall ensconcement of fluid from the capillary into the interstitial space. (A subset of diabulimia patients will already have developed renal damage from hyperglycemia, which results in urinary albumin excretion through microvascular and glomerular damage. Hypoalbuminemia through this mechanism eventualizes a decreased oncotic pressure, thus leaving excessive amounts of fluid in the extracellular space. Swelling in these patients is thus not entirely insulinogenic - they suffer from edema on a spectrum of severity even during extended periods of euglycemia/normoinsulinemia.)

Hypokalemia is one of the most dangerous reactions to insulin therapy, as it is an integral component of multiple physiological systems. Shocks of insulin administration drive excessive amounts of potassium from the extracellular fluid into the intracellular space by increasing activity of the sodium-potassium-ATP pump, which might induce dysfunction of both the cardiovascular and musculoskeletal systems.[5] Derangements in potassium levels pose a significant threat to cardiac rhythms and atrioventricular contractions, resulting in a variety of potentially life-threatening abnormalities such as ventricular tachycardia and fibrillation, AV blocks, and premature beats. Other adverse effects are transient muscle weakness and paralysis, which progresses from the lower to upper limbs if treated incorrectly. Hypokalemia also abets the phenomenon of sodium retention and edema potentiated by insulin. Reversal of low potassium levels results in increased natriuresis and subsequently decreased volume expansion.[3]

'Refeeding' functions will inevitably be activated – due to the deficiency of insulin sustained by the PWDb, the body will also have been starved of calories. Upon subjection to appropriate insulin doses, it stimulates the renin-angiotensin-aldosterone axis and other water-conserving systems as described above. This effect is typically seen with non-insulin-omitting eating disordered patients – especially those with anorexia nervosa – where a return to normal caloric intake can stimulate overzealous fluid retention. Indeed, the body strives to conserve fluids and electrolytes to such an extent that it qualifies as hypercompensation for the previous period of chronic hyperglycemic dehydration. Diabetic ketoacidosis is actually a state of secondary hyperaldosteronism, where the body senses the hyperglycemic osmotic diuresis and attempts to conserve volume as best as possible.[17] Some have speculated that the residual amount of aldosterone carrying over from the DKA state to that of euglycemia/normoinsulinemia also contributes to interstitial edema.

A majority of this insulinogenic fluid retention is reversible, although the PWDb must wait until the body equilibrates. The edema is generally protracted if the system has been starved of insulin for a longer interval. However, a proportion of weight gain following insulin treatment for diabulimia is actually permanent, and reflects 1.) glycogen repletion and the consequent hydration innate to increased liver storage of this molecule,[18] 2.) unexplained actions of insulin resulting in fat accumulation beyond what would be expected under otherwise normal circumstances, 3.) pharmacological side effects, and 4.) rehydration. Some patients concomitantly take prescriptions for psychiatric medications to treat the panic, anxiety, and depressant disorders which are strongly comorbid with diabulimia. Common side effects of these drugs are weight gain of unknown etiology, which the patient can experience following resumed 'compliance.'

Treatment of insulinogenic edema in Type I diabetes is still under pronounced debate. Diuretics such as furosemide, bumetanide, and spironolactone have been borderline effective on a case-by-case basis, as have insulin and salt restriction when such options were clinically acceptable.[4] However, prescription of diuretics in practice is not common because the metabolic state is already under such severe compromise – the PWDb is malnourished, centrally dehydrated, and hypotensive (despite the peripheral edema), and usually intentionally restricts fluid intake due to the sensation of bloating. Also, serum potassium might already be low due to the reinstitution of insulin, and diuretic administration (except spironolactone) would effect further potassium excretion and potential hypovolemia if not stringently monitored. Abnormal potassium levels are perilous for a multitude of reasons, and exacerbation with these medications is best avoided. In PWDbs whose condition has been so severe as to result in nephropathy, excretion of albumin in the urine is also aggravated by induced diuresis. These patients usually present with hypoalbuminemia and peripheral edema even before

3.) During the period of diabulimia, the brain assumes ketone bodies as its primary source of energy, secondary to the dangerously elevated levels of circulating ketones (which are also able to cross the blood-brain barrier).[21] As mentioned, it also progressively adopts hyperglycemia as a new baseline, despite decreased glucose usage secondary to elevated ketone perfusion. However, with abrupt reinstitution of insulin therapy, ketone production is inhibited and the brain is forced to utilize glucose once again for oxidation. Therefore, the patient's cognition will benefit from slow decreases in blood sugar, especially when combined with the a) concomitant reduction in ketone levels, b) neural readjustment to normal glucose levels.

4.) A gradual decrease in blood sugar is also protective against retinopathy and peripheral neuropathy, respectively. If these sequelae are already present, rapid decreases in blood sugar can result in diffuse neuropathic pain, which is consequently incapacitating. It can also cause acute swelling of muscles surrounding the orbit, leading to diplopia and other visual disturbances. Rapid correction of hyperglycemia also induces osmotic fluid shifts in the anterior and posterior chambers of the eye, which contributes towards blurred vision. .

Methods by which blood sugar and insulin are normalized can vary, but the dictum of gradual attenuation always takes precedence. If the patient's relative desire to commit to therapy is suboptimal, they might be convinced to maintain at least a basal insulin dose despite the continued absence of boluses or injections. This minimal amount of insulin will not effect dramatic modifications in the direction of euglycemia, but even a

---

insulin treatment onset – some so severe that diuretics have already been prescribed.

Patients themselves will attempt to defy the fluid retention by restricting their liquid intake, ingesting excessive amounts of caffeine (which is the most accessible natural diuretic through its inhibitory actions on endogenous anti-diuretic hormone), or herbal 'water pills.' These practices must be discouraged, as they only provoke the body to scavenge and retain more fluid; patients should rather drink proper amounts of fluid and refrain from excessive salt intake, so to slowly recompense for the hyperglycemic period of severe dehydration. As explained, endogenous physiological compensatory mechanisms sometimes prove overzealous, and it is best to let the body run its natural course in the case of insulin edema.

low-dose infusion will 1.) suppress ketone formation and 2.) inhibit the pathological increase in glucagon levels and subsequent exacerbation of hyperglycemia. On the other hand, if the patient demonstrates that they are amenable to therapy, the endocrinologist will generally aim for a stable 10 mg/dl decrease in blood glucose every week (anecdotal).

While the HbA1c is currently the best retrospective indicator of 2-3 month glycemic control and provides the most rapid results, it does not manifest immediate outcomes of treatment. Sometimes the endocrinologist needs to determine in a more expedient fashion whether their intervention is producing the desired results. To this end, some assess periodic fructosamine levels, which is a diagnostic marker with a much higher dynamic turnover, demonstrating changes within shorter periods. Ideal for periods of diabulimia recovery, it also provides positive reinforcement for the patients themselves, who are often derailed by the psychological discouragements that accompany treatment. Concrete evidence of improved glycemic numbers lends them again a nominal level of control that they perceive has been relinquished to the physician. This would not be quite as realistic with the *relatively* static HbA1c. (However, fructosamine, while supplying more frequent intermittent metabolic information, requires more time for laboratory analysis as it is performed on whole serum. Point-of-care HbA1c results, on the other hand, are available in less than 5 minutes – although admittedly less accurate than the serum test. The serum fructosamine is also generally considered less reliable a marker than the serum glycosylated hemoglobin.)

Initially, insulin dosing is largely relegated to the physician. However, as patients manifest improvement, they are granted progressive autonomy in this component of therapy. Various approaches are possible and should be maximized as per the patient's convenience. Insulin dosing and execution is often a burden, both mechanistically and psychologically, and presents a significant impediment to therapeutic compliance. Clinicians can ease this burden by recommending, as is appropriate for each PWDb, simpler insulin combinations or more basic insulin pump use. In combination with dietetic therapy, the PWDb learns to implement salutary nutritional intake and insulin doses to match, all of which are incrementally inculcated so as not to prompt relapse. The ultimate aim is not only to have patients independently dose themselves as per recommendation, but actually *desire* to do so. Results have demonstrated that the multidisciplinary approach is essential for achieving this goal.

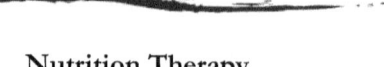

Nutrition Therapy

Nutrition represents a considerable constituent of the diabetes lifestyle; volumes can and have been penned on this subject alone. Here we will focus on the topic in pertinence to diabulimia, as it should be differentiated from both the general diabetes dietary regimen as well as the algorithms used to treat non-diabetic eating-disordered patients. Unfortunately, the nutritional guidelines on recuperation from these two pathologies are essentially antagonistic. Proper control – or a return to control – of Type I diabetes entails intense emphasis on understanding food and its glycemic/caloric properties; however, the therapy for disturbed eating attempts to gradually divert attention away from these materials. As a result, developing a course of therapy for PWDbs involves a different degree of complexity, especially considering the intimate relationship between the psychological and nutritional aspects of recovery.

The dietary treatment for diabulimia centers on a system termed "medical nutrition therapy (MNT)." Dieticians first comprehensively evaluate the patient's nutritional status, and then create an individually tailored intervention optimized for their lifestyle, dietary requirements, and personal preferences. Therapy continues longitudinally to ensure that 1.) the patient's medical and nutritional therapy are complementary, and also 2.) to implement any necessary changes warranted by shifts in either prognostic direction.

There are four basic goals of MNT for use in Type I diabetes, and each integrates within the overarching goal to preserve the patient's functionality.[6] The same principles apply to diabulimia. According to the American Diabetes Association, these are to:

1.) *Achieve maintained homeostasis in blood glucose, blood pressure, and lipid/lipoprotein ranges that have evidenced favorable outcomes for vascular and organ health.* For the PWDb, this includes not only gradual normalization of blood sugar in the short term, but also precautionary measures to prevent future relapse and progressive non-adherence with the prescribed course of therapy. Compromising this philosophy potentiates risk that the PWDb will feel overwhelmed, coerced, or encroached upon, and these mentalities are best avoided. The dietician must therefore be intimately aware of the individual's psychological inclinations and their particular reservations concerning food and eating, and communicate extensively with the psychiatric member of the diabetic team to ensure that they are aware of any factors likely to impede proper intake.

2.) *Prevent the incidence of complications resulting inevitably from poorly controlled glucose levels through dietary lifestyle modification.* This is a significant risk in diabulimia, as 'poorly controlled diabetes' is actually the intention of the illness, rather than a qualification to be pointedly avoided. The goal of MNT is to ensure that the PWDb can realizably modify nutritional intake during outpatient recovery without endangering their organs. This might include a focus on protein to maintain lower glucose levels, incorporation of fiber and low-glycemic carbohydrates to promote satiation while preventing insulin spiking, or moderate inclusion of fats to promote slower digestion and decreased appetite. The "rebound" effect should also be considered, namely that if the PWDb feels limited in one or multiple aspects of dietary intake, they might later over-consume that particular type of food (similar to the 'abstinence-violation effect'). This thereby negates the original intention, precipitating poor glucose control and even relapse.

3.) *Incorporate the patient's personal perspective, background, and history as pertaining to their willingness and ability to comply with the nutritional intervention.* Each patient with diabulimia has a unique ontology, which is a function of their familial/living dynamic, personality traits, and previous experiences with eating disorder/diabulimia course and recovery. The dietician is guaranteed to thwart themselves if they overlook these parameters as "softer" angles of a patient's case. Diabulimia is keenly psychological in orientation, and recovery efforts must carefully consider the bearing of each aspect on the patient's reaction to a dietary intervention.

4.) *Employ evidence-based nutritional therapy so as not to unnecessarily limit the patient from particular foods, thus detracting from their overall pleasure of eating.* This dictum is important for all the reasons enumerated above, but also for the nutritional element of diabulimia. For these patients who already generally possess an encyclopedic knowledge of food, unnecessarily limiting a specific dietary macronutrient sans scientific or clinical rationale is innately counterproductive. Professing, for example, that "eating high fructose corn syrup is bad" when there is no evidence to support such a claim might needlessly deprive the patient of an enjoyable entity, and likewise foil the dietician's attempt to elicit adherence.

5.) *In cases where complications have already crystallized, MNT must adopt the extra role of slowing their progress.* This is not an uncommon presentation in diabulimia, and must be integrated into the PWDb's nutritional plan. A patient suffering from diabulimia-induced nephropathy cannot be treated with the same approaches as a patient without microvascular sequelae. Their protein and electrolyte intake must be calibrated carefully so as not to subject the kidneys to additional stress and/or damage. The capacity to reverse some complications must be exploited to the fullest extent. Another issue, especially concerning restrictive PWDbs, is amenorrhea and compromised bone density acquired during the course of the illness (especially in adolescent patients where bone mineralization is at its peak). Studies have shown that nutritional rectification, rather than hormonal or vitamin supplementation, is more efficacious in restoring menstruation and potentially reversing osteopenia (age-, illness severity-, and bone location-dependent).[29]

The most important axiom arising from the multipronged approach towards diabulimia recovery (psychological and nutritional) is that of moderation. Elements of both regimens can be instituted into the same overall arrangement (despite their fundamental conflicts) as long they are in proper proportion. For example, consuming artificial sweeteners or 'diet' foods is discouraged for eating-disordered patients, but they are considered staple components of diabetes fare. The approach for a diabulimia patient, therefore, is to include these types of foods in a temperate fashion, thereby diminishing the risk of triggering adverse behaviors/outcomes on both fronts. The same concept applies to the intake of fat-rich foods. These are usually considered anathema for eating-disordered patients due to their dense caloric content, but nevertheless utilized by diabetes patients as an alternative to carbohydrates. Alternatively, they can be eaten in combination with carbohydrates to slow digestion and prevent hypoglycemic episodes provoked by spiking insulin.

It is also important to convey that there is nothing from which the PWDb is or will be prohibited from eating. One of the most unsavory features of 'recovery' entails a commencement of (or return to) ironclad abstinence from foods which they consider to be (or have been instructed are) 'unhealthy'/'undiabetic.' Not only is this comprehensively false, but also bolsters the role of these 'restricted' foods in provoking reversion into disordered eating. Such behavior includes bingeing, or even extending this dietary restraint into the elimination of other foods which were once considered normal. However, certain sacrifices are obligate: while the PWDb is not limited from any particular *type* of food, they must be willing to adjust quantities to optimally meet their caloric and nutritional requirements. The fact that they must also comply with insulin injections for their food choices goes without mention. (Obviously, a dietician would not issue similar freedoms to a non-eating-disordered or even non-diabetic subject – especially concerning saturated fats and sugars – as it neither guides the patient nor productively delineates boundaries for inevitably entitled 'cheating.' However, this approach is actually more effective for a refractory PWDb.)

Weight is not generally a priority during dietetic therapy for diabulimia, and in fact is not addressed explicitly with the patient due to its implications regarding detrimental mentations. During the initial stages of therapy (edema notwithstanding) patients will gain some weight due to dietary modifications and increased insulin. This is actually beneficial for some restrictive PWDbs, who can be severely clinically underweight. However, because it can be psychologically paralyzing for both restricting *and* bingeing patients, weight is monitored as a general vital sign by the clinician but not a variable disclosed during goal-oriented nutritional treatment. In the case that the patient would like to lose weight, the dietician and clinician will determine whether or not the patient's overall goal is legitimate/acceptable, and work with them to achieve the desired outcome.

Another perspective to be taken into consideration regarding dietary treatment for diabulimia is that concerning the PWDb's own knowledge of food. It cannot be impressed enough that eating-disordered patients – both insulin and non-insulin-omitting – usually have an exquisite knowledge of each number, value, and implication of food. Calories, carbohydrates, fat, fiber – they are exhaustively aware of everything, especially as it translates to their own body mass and allocation of weight. They know the exact location of particular foods to latitude and longitude, how much remains, and who is eating it. Many of them also know *exactly* how to dose insulin and are equally capable, if not more so, than other patients to produce normal HbA1c levels. Due to extended periods of negligence, some patients might need a 'refresher,' but a vast majority are startlingly proficient in terms of independent glycemic and dietary control. It is a common misconception that the dismal metabolic numbers during the first few months of therapy represent an inherent inability to execute the standard tasks of a Type I diabetic. (Contributions to poor glycemic control in this period also source from a brief period of "insulin refraction" during which the body's response to the hormone after reinstitution is highly unpredictable and often insensitive. This phenomenon is described later in the chapter, and does not preclude that the patient would know dosages under otherwise normal circumstances.)

Given this level of dietetic expertise regarding the specificity of their own insulin requirements, the observer might realistically question the advantage of a dietician in the recovery of a patient with diabulimia. After all, if the patient is expressly aware of everything the dietician will teach them, what is the possible purpose of reiteration? "There is nothing a Type I patient with diabulimia doesn't know – they are smarter than their dieticians *and* endocrinologists, so 'educating' them isn't going to do anything. You have to work through the issues in their head relating to eating and nutrition. You have to search out the reasons why they believe they aren't good enough for insulin. You have to be there alongside as they figure all of this out for themselves, as they go through the frightening initial stages of recovery, because if you don't foster a sense of trust then you're not helping anyone at all," states Scarlett Ramey, MS, RD, a dietician with extensive experience in the treatment of PWDbs.

As such, imbuing the patient with further instructions should not be the driving philosophy. Rather, the dietician (and diabetic team, for that matter), must seek to provide a supportive, reliable framework upon which the PWDb can begin to build a healthier lifestyle amenable to gradual physical – and more importantly – psychological recuperation. Although they might know their exact daily caloric requirements, the foods that fulfill it to the letter, and corresponding insulin doses, the patient is not generally well-versed in strategies of optimal recovery. They must be taught how to harness their own expertise so as to avoid psychosomatic subterfuge. Just as they are granted progressive autonomy over insulin administration, the patient is gradually allowed to create their own food plans as long as they demonstrate continued dedication towards appropriate qualitative/quantitative intake.

Here, we outline the major macronutrient groups (carbohydrates, protein, fat, and their sub-elements) within the context of diabulimia, and how dieticians can optimally integrate them into a nutritional intervention.

- *Carbohydrates*

Carbohydrates are arguably the most important dietary element for diabulimia patients –this is the macronutrient for which they must most frequently calculate insulin doses. (Under certain circumstances, protein and fat must also be accounted for with insulin; these will be discussed below.) Postprandial blood glucose peaks acutely without adequate amounts of insulin for carbohydrates, which is why it is important that the PWDb knows how to titrate each dose accordingly, as well as how to utilize this food group effactually in response to a hypoglycemic episode.

"Carbohydrate" as an overarching food group is nutritionally subdivided into "dietary fiber," sugar, and "other carbohydrates," namely what is listed on a standard nutrition label. Each component has different dynamics concerning their effect on blood sugar. The PWDb should maintain awareness of 1.) how each of these affects their insulin dosing, and 2.) that *all* can contribute to preservation of a healthy diet, weight, and HbA1c level.

Foods in general can be parsed according to their glycemic indices (GI), which are quantitative experimentally determined measures of the rate of absorption and digestion of the carbohydrate present in a particular food. Significant research has been devoted to this property in recent years given its implications for diabetic and overweight/obese patients. The rationale behind promoting low-glycemic carbohydrates lies in the fact that they do not induce a "spiking" blood sugar but rather a steady release of glucose that is salutary for diabetes management. Some longitudinal clinical trials have actually demonstrated reduced HbA1c levels through maintenance of a low-GI diet. Common examples of these foods are whole grains, nuts, green vegetables, and fructose from fruit sources; high-GI foods include white bread, potatoes, and glucose.

Low GI foods are useful to incorporate into all stages of diabulimia treatment. First, these types of foods tend to reduce the hunger pangs resulting from rapid increases in blood glucose and subsequent up-titration of insulin. One of the most common complaints upon reinstitution of insulin is the intense impetus to eat. These physical symptoms are highly inimical to maintaining a proper eating routine, and subsequently, metabolic control. Also, low GI foods lower the insulin necessary for the initial phases of recovery, during which many PWDb's experience brief to extended periods of insulin 'refraction' (their bodies manifest decreased changes for the same dose of insulin than that of previous euglycemic periods.) This is secondary to 1.) downregulation of the insulin receptor on somatic cells following protracted exposure to toxic levels of glucose, 2.) orthoglycemia in some patients effects an increase in renal insulin clearance due to kidney proximal tubular damage, necessitating larger doses to maintain the plasma concentration.[11] These peculiarities complicate insulin dosing, frustrate the dietetic endeavors of diabulimia recovery, and potently aggravate the syndrome of diabetes discouragement ("burnout"). The benefits of these foods must therefore be explored on a case-by-case basis, but not emphasized at the expense of dietary variety. While low-GI foods might improve metabolic control, it is inaccurate and even detrimental for a patient to believe that eating them at the expense of higher glycemic foods is the ultimate goal of diabetic MNT concerning carbohydrates.

High-GI foods are very useful for hypoglycemic episodes as they rapidly normalize the blood sugar. Hypoglycemia is a major precipitating factor of disordered eating in diabetic patients, as it physiologically induces an elevated appetite. As a consequence, patients experiencing low blood sugar 1.) overcompensate in terms of carbohydrate intake, or 2.) consume foods that are unsuited for raising glucose levels, and later omit insulin for such an episode. Therefore, the patient should know the specific high-GI foods most optimized for rectifying hypoglycemia, and maintain them in appreciable vicinity.

Sugars are a rather nuanced subset of carbohydrates as well, especially in regards to the PWDb. Unfortunately, sugars as a dietary entity are vilified in the public eye, impressions which many PWDbs are guaranteed to have internalized. The danger sugars pose to weight loss, dieting, and diabetes lies not in their inherent nutritional properties but in their remarkable predilection to be abused – a feature highlighted only by their comparably greater palatability. This effect is further bolstered by the reigning falsehood that "Type I diabetic patients are not allowed to eat sugar," which is perhaps one of the most heinous misconceptions in circulation. Unfortunately, some diabetic patients become so inculcated with this urban myth such that they pathologically deprive themselves of sugar-containing carbohydrates, leading frequently to rebound overconsumption and consequent development of eating disorders/diabulimia ('abstinence-violation' principle).

Given this environment, the dietician must be extremely wary of rhetoric pertaining to sugar, and focus on underscoring moderation as a universal application. As long as 1.) adequate amounts of insulin are allotted for their consumption, and 2.) their ingestion does not produce adverse effects (excessive weight gain, compromises in other food groups, psychosomatic instability), limiting "sugary foods" is inappropriate.

Fiber is generally parsed into soluble and insoluble groups. Soluble fiber dissolves in water and is construed into metabolically usable byproducts in the gastrointestinal tract. It has long been a target of cardiovascular and gastrointestinal research secondary to its hypothesized role in cholesterol and lipid reduction. Insoluble fiber, on the other hand, remains metabolically inert through the course of its passage through the body, adding bulk to the stools through absorption and holding of water. Soluble fiber is present in oats, apples, psyllium husks, and green vegetables; insoluble fiber can be found in lentils, beans, berries, and bran.

Fiber provides multiple benefits when incorporated into a PWDb's MNT plan. For reasons described in Chapter 7, serum lipid panels are sometimes abnormal, and raise concern regarding prevention of coronary heart disease and other sequelae for which the insulin-dependent diabetic is at risk. Although these usually self-rectify to a certain extent following replacement of adequate insulin, a diet complementary to homeostasis of healthy cholesterol – here, through inclusion of soluble fiber – should be underscored. Next, fibrous foods generally have lower overall calorie:gram ratios compared to their starchier peers, providing considerable dietary bulk without precipitating weight gain if consumed in relatively greater amounts. As mentioned, somatic (not just psychogenic) "cravings" are typical of insulin therapy reinstatement. The PWDb might attempt to ignore or suppress these signals due to their sensitivity towards caloric repercussion, which is detrimental to the efficacy of dietary interventions. Fiber-rich foods counteract increased appetite by providing essential vitamins, minerals, and also a powerful source of satiation. Lastly, insoluble fiber, being indigestible roughage – does not require insulin – it is subtracted from the total number of carbohydrates for calculation of a bolus[7] if it is approximately greater than five grams per meal. *Soluble* fiber, being metabolized, requires about half the insulin the patient would require were it a standard carbohydrate. Albeit marginally, these properties reduce the overall required insulin, preventing spiking, as well as potential reduction in edema during the initial phase of therapy.

Artificial sweeteners and sugar substitutes are potentially problematic in that they, unlike other carbohydrate subcategories, intrinsically straddle the realms of eating disorders and diabetes. This feature is attributed to their ability to eliminate/dampen the caloric repercussions of carbohydrates with minimal/no concessions in taste. This renders them vulnerable to abuse, and indeed are sometimes ingested in excess of safety, or as inappropriate alternatives to proper nutrition. PWDbs might exploit them to further curtail their caloric intake and thus enhance weight loss. Upon restoration of proper metabolic control, however, both restricting and bingeing diabulimic patients are prone to misusing these products. They provide a placebo flavor which mitigates the self-imposed limitation of sugars and all their caloric ramifications.

Nonetheless, artificial sweeteners/sugar substitutes are practical incorporations for both normal diabetic and diabulimic patients. They require little to no insulin if consumed in appropriate amounts. For example, instead of calculating the amount of insulin required for the few teaspoons of sugar appended to a mug of coffee, a patient might stir in a moderate amount of Splenda,® Equal,® or Truvia,® and efficiently eliminate this extra burden.[11] Palatability is a possible impediment, but many brands have been carefully gauged to optimally mimic the flavor of real sugar. The dietician should emphasize that these "sugar substitutes" must not replace a normal level of carbohydrates. Rather, they should bolster the advantages of insulin regimen simplification as well as provide balanced alternatives to excessive sugar in the overall dietary intake.

We will reinforce, especially in the light of common belief, that carbohydrates are injurious to neither diabetes control nor weight control. They represent a crucial component of any dietetic diabetes intervention, providing essential fuels for the body and brain, a specific subset of micronutrients, and prevention/correction of hypoglycemic episodes. Their dietary incorporation is crucial for any PWDb undergoing both the initial phases of recovery as well as longitudinal maintenance of metabolic control. All carbohydrates (sugars, fiber, and starches) should be incorporated according to the proportion *and* purpose for which they are most likely to mollify the psychological/physical travails of continued therapy.

- *Proteins*

Proteins are also an important part of MNT for Type I diabetes, and their incorporation into the dietary plan for patients with normal renal function is generally no different from that of the normal population (15-20% of total caloric intake). Renal compromise, however, should always be considered when present. The glomerular filtration rate (GFR) of Type I diabetic patients is initially elevated even under conditions of euglycemia (due to selective hyaline arteriosclerosis of the efferent glomerular arteriole, which increases the capillary pressure filtration). Increased GFR in turn leads to 1) mesangial ingrowth, leading to formation of pathognomonic

---

[11]   Some sugar substitutes are not as simple and must be highlighted for the equanimity and education of the PWDb. These include the sugar alcohols (e.g. maltitol and lactitol), commonly encountered in "Lo-carb" or "Atkins" prepackaged foods. Contrary to popular diet culture, these *are* absorbed within the gastrointestinal tract and metabolized. They therefore possess 1.) discernable caloric value and 2.) also require insulin due to their structural homologies with pure sugar. This must be accounted for when aiding the patient in deciding how best to incorporate sugar substitutes into the new dietary plan.

hyaline glomerular bodies known as Kimmelstein-Wilson nodules, 2) elevated filtration of proteins, which must consequently be reabsorbed in the renal tubules. This hyperabsorption of proteins consequently induces inflammatory cascades culminating in fibrosis of kidney parenchyma. High protein intake further advances hyperfiltration especially in patients with decreased renal function.[8] The danger of precipitating renal damage is substantial if the PWDb attempts to surpass certain dietary delineations. Considering the detriment they have already imposed on their kidneys through intentionally perpetuated hyperglycemia, PWDbs are much more likely to have some level of renal damage. Discretion is hence required when 'prescribing' levels of protein intake.

This is not to imply that proteins cannot be utilized during outpatient nutritional treatment for diabulimia – in fact, they entail multiple benefits for both the diabetes and eating disorder components of diabulimia. They rarely require insulin (unless consumed in atypically large amounts), which streamlines insulin dosing and aids in suppressing the initial phases of insulinogenic edema. Also, a significant proportion of protein's innate caloric value is dedicated towards digestive metabolism by virtue of its high thermogenic content. In order to convert them into tissue-utilizable form, the body must expend substantial energy to catabolize whole proteins into individual amino acids. These amino acids enter respective energy-producing machineries through glucogenesis, ketogenesis, or as substrates for synthetic reactions. During this extensive processing, the body's metabolic rate is appreciably (but only temporarily) increased. Also, whole proteins foster satiety, compared to isocaloric diets comprised of higher proportions of carbohydrates and fats.[9] Protein can delay gastric release, which signals repletion, and slows absorption of some carbohydrates. This 'synthetic low-GI' effect shields from hypoglycemia-induced hunger.

As such, proteins have been lionized as the savior for weight-loss tribulations, and assimilated in ever-increasing dietary magnitudes. Also beneficial for diabulimia therapy, they allay hunger triggers in two ways. They 1.) support a decreased volume of caloric intake following insulin reinstitution due to appetite repletion, and 2.) decrease the effective circulating insulin concentration, thereby attenuating its direct stimulation of the body's 'hunger' apparatus (protein does not usually require insulin bolusing).

Due to these aforementioned benefits (elevation of metabolic rate/satiation levels and abridgment of insulin doses), the PWDb might attempt to consume this macronutrient at the inappropriate expense of carbohydrate and fat, due to either fear of hunger or a recurrent fixation on weight loss and caloric negation. Compromising the nutritional benefits of other macronutrients to exploit the advantages of protein is improper even while under the umbrella of outpatient normoinsulinemia. It is the dietician's role to provide proper guidance, rationale, and encouragement regarding a level of intake befitting the patient's history, current renal status, and psychological status/progression.

- *Fats*

Fats are likely to affect the eating disordered PWDb's psyche and must be treated with genuine sensitivity. Along with carbohydrates, fats have historically been disparaged as antagonistic to health and weight loss, but these simplistic impressions hold no scientific corroboration and in fact are harmful if adopted and implemented as fact. Fats and their metabolites are essential for brain health, heat production, organ integrity, and energy storage; deficiencies in any constituent consequent to dietary restriction can be severely debilitating to physical and mental acuity. Individuals with eating disorders, especially restrictive (and some purging) PWDbs, have a penchant for eschewing this food group – if not for the caloric density, then for the misconception that direct consumption automatically causes weight gain, i.e. "eating fat makes you fat." For these reasons, the dietician must understand, in tandem with the team's mental health professional, the particular reservations that the PWDb harbors concerning fat and its ramifications, and address those concerns while incorporating this macronutrient into the overall dietary construction.

Similar to carbohydrates, fats are divided for the purpose of the dietician into categories encountered on an average food label. These are saturated, trans, polyunsaturated, and monounsaturated fats. The provisos regarding each subcategory are generally not specific to the PWDb (as opposed to the classifications of carbohydrates) – the latter two are lauded as beneficial for the heart, and should be consumed in greater amounts to rectify high cholesterol levels. Per contra, saturated and trans fats are considered harmful to vascular health, and are generally present in the highest proportions in 'junk foods such as chips, cookies, cakes, and meats. Tact is important when explaining to the PWDb (especially the bingeing subtype) how they can productively integrate adequate quantities of these foods, without emphasizing the limitations. Previously bingeing PWDbs will resent that they used to be able to ingest these palatable 'junk and 'comfort' foods sans weight or cardiovascular repercussions. As such, exercising portion control will likely pose some challenges.

Despite particular stipulations, 'fats' as a general dietary concept for the PWDb cannot be overlooked. Fats postpone gastric emptying (similar to proteins, but with a greater delay) by stimulating the release of the hormone cholecystokinin from the small intestine to allow more time for intestinal digestion and absorption. As described previously, mechanical and biochemical effects of fat hold numerous benefits for the PWDb. First, when combined with other ingredients, fat promotes a greater sensation of satiety for meals of isocaloric value. Second, the delay in gastric emptying applies to all foods eaten in tandem, which can be helpful for insulin dosing if fat represents a minor part of the overall meal. (Patients with gastroparesis are obviously an exception.) Carbohydrates especially are released into the bloodstream at a slightly slower rate, preventing unanticipated blood sugar swings.[12]

- *Calories*

There is some debate surrounding the traditional 'calories in – calories out' equation ascribed to by dieticians and weight-loss experts the world over. Some argue that the 'type' of calorie (protein, type of fat, type of carbohydrate) and overall proportion of macronutrients creates internal discrepancies between the total energy harnessed by the body; others maintain that the timing of intake determines the extent of caloric burning. However, these variables should not be unduly emphasized in terms of the

---

[12] However, when fats constitute a majority of the meal, they cause whatever carbohydrates are ingested simultaneously to absorb inordinately late, necessitating the use of what are termed "square" or "dual" wave boluses on the pump. Insulin dosing for fats, more so than that for proteins, is a complicated and highly imprecise science, varying distinctly between individuals.

overall caloric counseling for a PWDb, as this engenders an environment ripe for fixation on numbers and weight. Considering that these were possible etiologies of diabulimia in the first place, dwelling conspicuously – however innocently – on any aspect of this disordered-eating-sensitive topic is not recommended.

As such, proposing specific numbers in terms of daily caloric intake – such as basal and resting metabolic rates – is avoided in favor of approximations.[13] This approach precludes unfavorable mentation provoked by the existence of an exact caloric ceiling and/or basement. Prescribing a narrow caloric window generates 1.) sensations of entrapment, eliciting frustration, dissatisfaction, disillusionment, and ultimately potential relapse, or 2.) obsessive adherence to that particular value, such that aberrance inspires impressions of failure. These impressions threaten to deconstruct the severe discipline that the PWDb has cultivated in the period of recovery, which, needless to say, is another pathway of regression into diabulimia once again.

Provided the psychological underpinnings concerning perfectionism, weight control, and caloric cognition – and especially as all of these relate to tight glucose management – the PWDb might swing to another end of the eating spectrum. Compared to the unfavorable intake patterns practiced during the insulin-omitting period, they can become inordinately focused upon optimizing their diets. Exacerbating this is the necessity for tight glucose management during the sustained course of recovery, which

---

[13]   There are various equations utilized to calculate basal and resting metabolic rates, but these are also burdened with some imprecision – comparisons between randomly elected algorithms differ more than is statistically warranted. The Harris-Benedict is by far the most commonly utilized for research purposes. Although it is almost never used at face value in the clinical setting, it underlies many of the approximations used by dieticians and physicians. These are "ballparks" for the PWDb, and generally range from 1500-2500 kcal per day. It should function secondary to the inclusion of adequate macronutrient and micronutrient allotments. If anything, erring should be on the side of higher intake, as one criticism of metabolic rate equations is their propensity to underestimate the true value necessary for providing total micromolecular nutrition. The equanimity and productivity of the patient should be referenced, ensuring that their caloric intake grants them adequate levels of mental and physical energy.

necessarily promotes the concept of proper eating and nutrition. As such, the former PWDb might develop an obsession with 'nutritionally sound' food consumption, such that proper nutrition is counterintuitively compromised. At the expense of a micronutritionally varied diet, the patient will elect foods which at face value are considered 'healthy' (by public or medical definition, or otherwise) and consume them out of proportion, consequently denying themselves other selections. "Orthorexia nervosa," is the unofficial term for this preoccupation regarding 'correct' calories. Fixation upon healthy food intake is dangerous when extrapolated to extreme levels, due to the compromise the practice imposes on other food groups. Even when nutritional intake is adequate under this "orthorexic" umbrella, these food-related obsessions and their progressive psychological integration nevertheless prove to be injurious. The PWDb in recovery finds that they must deal with the mental onslaught of caloric/nutritional rectification, weight gain, as well as the paradox of having to focus on food (for diabetes management) while trying to correct any deviant mentation (for eating disorder management). When all pathological escape routes are blocked (e.g., purging and/or caloric restriction) during the recovery process, the PWDb desperately attempts to reclaim control by another 'normal' avenue – here, 'correct' eating. What commences as an innocuous diet quietly transforms into one detrimentally fixated on the righteousness of ingested food. The PWDb must internalize from treatment onset that certain otherwise-vilified foods (and also caloric intake) are not 'correct' or 'incorrect.' Rather, any and all can be incorporated in reasonable proportions for healthy diet fulfillment.

- *Alcohol*

Alcohol consumption must be addressed as it has ramifications on both blood sugar as well as disordered eating. First, it can induce hypoglycemia in both moderate to excessive intake. The metabolism of ethanol in the liver leads to an increased protonation of the NAD molecule, which diverts the conversion of pyruvate to lactate instead of acetyl CoA, thereby preventing its progression to the aerobic Krebs cycle. It also reroutes oxaloacetate to malate, stalling the Krebs cycle and shuttling acetyl CoA towards production of ketones. Both diversions 1.) inhibit gluconeogenesis and 2.) direct the products of metabolism towards fatty acid synthesis. Alcohol can also distort the metabolism of glucose itself, rendering the patient prone to unpredictable and refractory glycemic readings for a consequently indeterminate period of time. This is especially problematic in patients who elect to drink on an empty stomach in an effort to enhance absorption and hence the onset of alcoholic effects.

Alcohol also has implications for disordered eating. The nutritional labeling of alcohol is highly inconsistent, with multiple laws regulating the requirements of alcohol content, additives, and calories across various types of spirits (pure ethanol contains 7 kilocalories per gram, as compared to 9 for fats and 4 for carbohydrates and protein). It is nevertheless generally regarded as an energy-dense liquid. Patients with anorexic proclivity, or those quantifying calories, will intentionally consume fewer portions of solid food in order to drink greater quantities of alcohol (thus maintaining a predetermined caloric ceiling), which is a very dangerous methodology considering the hypoglycemic effects described above. By eating less *per os*, the patient has already primed themselves for low blood glucose, which is only compounded by ethanol's inhibitory effects on the liver.

PWDbs with cyclical binge-purge patterns will intentionally overconsume alcohol to induce vomiting, which creates a caloric deficit (or simply neutrality) through expulsion of the ingested ethanol. Concomitant with these intentional alcoholic binge episodes, some patients will also ingest excessive quantities of solid food, knowing that the liqueur's emetic effects will later aid in its pathological expulsion. Binges can also be involuntary, induced by stress or depression (as is frequently manifest during recovery). Alcohol is a powerful coping mechanism, and PWDbs with a history of prior alcohol dependence/abuse, or a tendency towards substance addictive behavior might use it to assuage anxiety regarding weight gain, eating, or other adverse cognition. Of note, alcohol abuse and eating disorders are also highly comorbid, with the causality putatively bidirectional.

PWDbs should be counseled regarding the hazards of this substance in both the long- and short-term. As alcohol is a ubiquitous substance central to many social gatherings, diplomatic verbalization is necessary to impress that it is not 'forbidden' (unless clinically contraindicated). As always, averting acute hypoglycemia must be prioritized, as it not only prevents 1.) immediate risk to the patients consciousness and physical stability, but also 2.) a psychosomatic spearhead for binge episodes. Taking precautions such as prophylactic snacking prior to drinking alcohol, carrying a source of glucose, and monitoring blood sugar levels closely is judicious. As events touting sources of alcohol are generally more likely to occur later in the day, the PWDb should be sure to test prior to sleeping to protect from nocturnal hypoglycemia. Of course, it goes without saying that moderation of alcohol intake must also be underscored.

Exercise

Exercise is beneficial for both the body and the brain, and is recommended in many therapeutic settings. As described, the patient might be wary of eating adequately for fear of adopting a particular body image – exercise alleviates some of this anxiety by opening a healthy avenue towards weight control. Burning calories, decreasing appetite, increasing metabolic rate, building lean muscle, sustaining energy, prompting endogenous endorphin and opioid release – the benefits of exercise in regards to body perception/morphology are replete. Not only does it aid in weight control, but also plays a role in the maintenance of blood glucose. Exercise makes the muscles more sensitive to insulin both in the short term (during the immediate episode of exercise) as well as longitudinally (the body, even during periods of rest, will require less insulin for the same degree of glycemic normalization than would be present without regular exercise patterns). Eating post-exercise also does not increase blood glucose to the same magnitude, as the liver appropriates and shuttles circulating glucose towards formation of glycogen shelved for the next session of exercise, hypoglycemia, or starvation.

Unfortunately, exercise can be similarly exploited and manipulated for the purposes of weight control. Excessive exercise, similar to insulin omission, is considered to be an inappropriate compensatory behavior in both anorexia nervosa and bulimia nervosa. If the patient does not receive a proper course of psychiatric treatment in tandem with physiological stabilization, the cognitive issues precipitating the disordered behaviors remain at large – beyond the patient's control – and channel themselves into other detrimental behaviors. For example, the PWDb might manage to internalize, accept, and implement the concept that insulin omission is *not* an option under any circumstance, but still harbor abnormal thoughts concerning the matters of body shape and mass. These consequently manifest in improper behaviors originating as either 1.) acceptable, namely exercise and proper nutrition, which then become excessive/"orthorexic" or 2.) inappropriate, such as vomiting and unnecessary laxative/diuretic use.

Exercise, contrary to popular belief, does require insulin under certain circumstances (discussed below). If the PWDb still manifests trepidation or antagonism towards proper insulin dosing, this line of treatment must be placed on hiatus or abandoned. Engaging in marginally strenuous physical activity while hyperglycemic is highly dangerous, and to do so while hyperketotic is nigh toxic. The American Diabetes Association recommends that focused exercise intentionally be foregone if blood sugar levels are greater than 250 mg/dl with ketones, or above 300 mg/dl without ketones. These levels are chosen less for their absolute magnitude than for what their relative amounts represent in terms of an insulin deficiency. If exercise is undertaken during these circumstances, disproportionate amounts of fatty acids are oxidized for fuel, leading to development of (or an exacerbated) ketonemia.

There are two fundamental divisions of exercise which can overlap depending on the respective level of exertion. These activities are aerobic (jogging, cycling, basketball), and anaerobic (most types of weightlifting, sprinting, plyometrics). Biochemically, aerobic exercise breaks apart glucose and uses oxygen as a terminal electron receptor in creating energy. Anaerobic exercise, on the other hand, shuttles glucose towards formation of lactic acid in the absence of oxygen.[14]

---

14   Glucogenic energy sources from two main locations during aerobic and anaerobic exercise in a diabetic patient – the gastrointestinal tract, and the liver. Carbohydrates ingested pre-workout are absorbed into the bloodstream via the small intestine. During aerobic exercise in a patient with intact beta cells, muscle contractions trigger a signaling cascade that *partially* dampens insulin release, which in turn allows glucagon to signal hepatocytes and striated muscle cells to commence glycogenolysis. The net production of glucose increases, but the tissue utilization of glucose also increases simultaneously through 1.) increased peripheral blood flow and more efficient delivery of insulin 2.) stimulating, *even in the absence of insulin*, translocation of more GLUT4 transporters to the cell membrane. (GLUT4 is the glucose portal in striated muscle cells, and does not generally appear at the cell

The processes undergone during aerobic, low-intensity exercise go awry in a Type I patient if not monitored closely with exogenous insulin and glucose testing. Without insulin to permit glucose entrance into muscle cells, glucagon levels are elevated and still stimulate glycogenolysis. This exercise-released glucose accumulates in the bloodstream, leading to hyperglycemia and premature exhaustion; the body also resorts to fat catabolism to generate the requisite energy, leading to ketone formation. On the other hand, if a diabetic patient eats a meal, doses herself an adequate amount for the carbohydrate content, and then decides to go for an impromptu bike ride, she will in all likelihood have a hypoglycemic episode. (This does not occur in a non-diabetic patient because insulin levels are more intimately calibrated – the beta-cells release insulin as they 'see' glucose. In other words, as the blood sugar incrementally increases or decreases, the level of secreted insulin will wax and wane in proportion; the beta-cells do not eject in one fell dose, as compared with an exogenously administered injection/bolus – one of the many stipulations concerning insulin therapy. During exercise, islet cells will immediately sense any

---

membrane in appreciable amounts sans insulin or exercise). In both diabetic and non-diabetic patients under exercise conditions, insulin enhances this response by forcing larger quantities of intracellular GLUT4 transporters to insert at the cell surface, thereby allowing more glucose to enter cells than what would be expected under conditions of rest.[22] Thus, in a normal individual, there is no outstanding increase in blood glucose levels, as the glucose production is similar to peripheral glucose utilization under regulation by the insulin:glucagon ratio.[24]

Anaerobic or "high-intensity" exercise is a marginally different matter, involving the actions of dramatically increased circulating catecholamine levels (epinephrine and norepinephrine). These hormonal neurotransmitters have more directly potent effects than the insulin:glucagon ratio during anaerobic activity by powerfully stimulating muscle and liver glycogenolysis while simultaneously antagonizing muscle glucose uptake and insulin release. Net glucose production is thereby rendered greater than peripheral glucose utilization. (Compare this to aerobic exercise, in which these two variables are almost equivalent in the presence of basal insulin.) Hyperglycemia ensues even in a normal patient for the interval of anaerobic activity. Fortunately, this elevated plasma glucose is neutralized during recovery by elevated levels of insulin rescued from inhibition by the post-exercise decrease in circulating catcholamines.[23]

Obviously, this insulin-generating response is absent in diabetic patients, and unfortunately why anaerobic exercise actually leaves a trail of hyperglycemia in its wake. The amount of insulin injected usually underestimates the catecholamine-perpetuated glucose accumulation, as patients will only bolus for the amount of food that they might have ingested prior – or even *underdose*, anticipating the 'exercise effect.'

trending hypoglycemia, suppress an already enfeebled secretion of insulin, and upregulate glucagon to maintain the plasma glucose at a stable level.)

Although a diabetic patient might incorporate previous or projected aerobic exercise into calculating their insulin dose, they still run the risk for hyperglycemic excursions. They should always ensure the proximity of a glucose source during a bout of exercise or sports game to counteract possible lows. Liver glycogen stores are also depleted post-exercise, necessitating carbohydrates to replenish the plasma glucose that hepatocytes and striated muscles consume for glycogenesis. It is also generally recommended that individuals ingest a few extra calories after moderate-intensity exercise in order to antagonize the muscle catabolism concomitant with oxidation of glucose or fat.

As mentioned previously, recovering PWDbs who still harbor abnormal thoughts and emotions towards weight/shape/food are at elevated risk for the diabetes-related toxicities of exercise, even in the absence of disproportionate exertion. Carbohydrate and caloric replenishment post-exertion are nigh required for a Type I diabetic in order to avoid acute hypoglycemia as the liver and muscles scavenge glucose from the bloodstream. Many PWDbs or eating disordered patients engage in exercise primarily to lose weight (as opposed to health benefit, increased vitality, mood improvement, or enjoyable recreation). Such an impetus, while valid, can impinge upon proper nutritional supplementation prior to, during, and after exercise. Ingesting calories and then burning them (or vice versa – burning calories followed by post-exercise caloric replenishment) during exercise are to the eating disordered patient fundamentally at odds, leading to sometimes severe hypoglycemia and diminished energy.

Engaging in high-intensity exercise can prove beneficial for the PWDb but only if executed properly and with appropriate motivation. This entails 1.) pre-exercise: proper dosing of insulin and perhaps caloric supplementation, 2.) intra-exercise: perception of hypoglycemic symptoms and responding appropriately, and 3.) post exercise: blood glucose monitoring and caloric/glucose supplementation (even if glycemic levels are normal). Anaerobic exercise, such as weightlifting or sprinting, involves dynamic muscle turnover, the equilibrium of which depends on hormonal activity as well as nutritional status. Both insulin *and* calories are required to avoid sacrificing lean tissue through exercise-induced catabolism without compensatory anabolism. (Insulin is the consummate anabolic hormone, and combined with appropriate calories will restore glycogen reservoirs as well as lean tissue broken down by bouts of intense physical activity.) The PWDb might undertake anaerobic exercise for the directed purpose of losing weight, and while this is acutely accomplished, they actually risk long term weight gain due to ramifications of relinquished muscle mass (consequences of which are a decrease in both resting metabolic rate and energy). Exercising anaerobically for extended periods of time is also destructive, and some PWDbs will do so despite exhaustion. These consequences illustrate the importance of appropriate motivation and mental status for physical activity – if the recovering PWDb exercises for the purpose of "shedding pounds quickly" or without proper relationships with food and general diabetes management, they risk 1.) deviant glycemic values, 2.) long-term weight gain and exacerbation of body/shape concern, and/or 3.) inability to continue this beneficial activity.

Psychiatric and Psychological Treatment

Psychotherapy transcends the other overarching variables of diabulimia therapy (insulin and nutrition), as each of these, by default, factors into the mental status. It is, perhaps arguably, the most crucial component of the recovery process. Diabetic teams can correct blood sugar and energy intake and send the patient packing, but if the underlying psychopathology of the eating disorder is ignored then both clinician and patient will inevitably find themselves back at square one. It must be mentioned that a majority of the following information is derived from anecdotal evidence, and has not been comprehensively validated by clinical studies.

Effective outpatient methodologies involved in treatment of eating disorders include cognitive-behavioral therapy (CBT), family-based therapy (FBT), interpersonal psychotherapy (IPT), self-directed treatment, and/or pharmacological interventions. Some physicians will maintain that diabulimia can be treated as they would any other eating disorder, and this is a practical approach especially given the lack of concrete research data pertaining to the condition. However, there are some qualitative problems with this philosophy. Insulin omission is diabetes-specific, and these patients' baseline mental statuses are dramatically different than that of the general eating-disordered population. Cognitions (especially those concerning food) considered pathological in a non-diabetic are regarded as completely normal in a diabetic individual due to the nutritional/pharmacologic features of the illness. Therefore, it is essential to address the issue of insulin omission *specifically*, rather than approaching diabulimia from a 'holistic' purging mechanism angle. Correcting the mental issues from which the eating disorder derives in order to attenuate its symptomatic manifestations (viz., purging in general), is still a highly valid and efficacious method. However, it compromises full cognitive recovery by failing to tackle the specific issues relating to diabetes-induced disordered eating and insulin omission.

Official psychotherapy generally only commences after the PWDb's blood sugar levels are ostensibly reduced (usually to around 200-250 mg/dl) for an appropriate period of time. Above 250 mg/dl, patients simply do not possess optimal intellectual capacity – hyperglycemia fosters a state of distraction, confusion, rational fallacy, and mental fatigue. This status is obviously counterproductive for the clinician attempting to address perceptive abnormalities. Patients with chronic diabulimia, having plodded through hyperglycemia for extended periods, will actually – to both themselves and their clinicians – appear to have full cognitive capacity. This phenomenon is attributed to both physiological and psychological factors: 1.) the body and brain compensate for the elevated blood sugars, ultimately adjusting their functions to match the chronic hyperosmolarity, and 2.) the patient, recognizing the cerebral symptoms of hyperglycemia, works even harder to override them in a type of temporary 'therapeutic denial' by taking active stances against distraction and working/short-term memory losses (primarily through awareness-correction mechanisms). However, *despite* extenuations and professions to the contrary, patients' a.) insights into their condition, b.) mental statuses, and c.) attention spans under higher blood sugar levels are not ideal for the rigor of psychotherapy.

During this treatment window, the patient can undergo an "educational" type of counseling. This phase is designed to warn, equip, and underscore benefits of diabetes treatment. First and foremost, the patients are reminded that their brain is not at optimal functional capacity, and that lowering glycemic values will result in improvement on all fronts, both physical and psychological. More quotidian incentives should also be emphasized; they might actually be more powerful than the conventional psychiatric methods described later, simply by virtue of their accessibility and strong resonance. They are readily accessible sources of positive reinforcement that do not require medical personnel, and should be relayed to the patient as encouragement and impetus to life with insulin and normoglycemia. "Good health," as both an overarching concept as well as its encompassing minutiae, is a useful goal to impress upon the patient:

- ➤ Improved mental function – less confusion/lack of focus, ability to engage in meaningful conversation
- ➤ Improved memory – fewer amnestic symptoms from chronic hyperglycemia
- ➤ Less anxiety from deceptive methods or appearance of the next random/predictable complication to result from a lack of insulin
- ➤ Recurrence of, or improved menses and sexual function – capacity to have children and intimate relationships
- ➤ Pregnancy – maintenance of a safe fetal environment. Patients have been able to "quit diabulimia cold-turkey" at pregnancy onset in order to protect the fetus from intrauterine hyperglycemic damage, and some have been able to continue their normoglycemic patterns of behavior postpartum.
- ➤ Energy – ability to participate in normal activities
- ➤ Hair growth – reversal of malnourishment-induced follicle loss/friability
- ➤ Better skin – hydration and vitamins are supplied to this organ concomitant with insulin reinstitution

In general, many abnormal somatic processes are suppressed after return to nominal eu-glycemia/insulinemia and proper nutrition. This fact should be capitalized during both the pre-, intra-, and post-psychotherapy phases of diabulimia treatment.

During this pre-psychotherapy phase, the patient is also warned about 'monkey wrenches' that are almost guaranteed to present during treatment. Edema is one of the most significant. As described, this manifests as central or peripheral swelling in a vast majority (although differentially expressed among the diabulimia population), and is a cruel phenomenon that powerfully antagonizes any desire to fully convalesce. It is essential, especially during this period, that patients constantly be reassured that the ostensible weight gain is only transient fluid retention, and in many cases totally reversible. Even though the patient might have previously attempted self-medication with insulin and already be sensitive to edema, validation of this reversibility is very important as it is *never* a self-evident projection. This reassurance will serve to be a substantial leap towards recuperation, as this initial shock induces a substantial number of relapses.

Patients are also cautioned concerning these relapses into insulin omission (or other purging mechanisms). Regressive behavior occurs frequently and as such is actually considered a standard component of the longitudinal recovery process. These acute or extended transgressions can be interpreted as incapacity or failure, which is both immediately and chronically demoralizing. Patients might begin to believe that recovery is impossible and failure inevitable given the number of times that they have foundered, leading to entrapment within this self-fulfilling prophecy. Such cognitions can exacerbate the recurrence of insulin omission such that 1.) the current episode is extended, possibly leading to full relapse and 2.) thresholds for future recurrence and relapse are lowered. Equipping the patient with a positive perspective concerning relapse can dramatically improve their chances of recovery, especially during earlier stages when the "memories" of diabulimia are still in proximity.

Psychological therapy itself is highly complex and individually tailored – it is impossible within our scope to describe each of the various treatment permutations. However, it is useful to be familiar with the following general concepts.

An important aspect of psychological treatment (overlapping with nutritional intervention) is normalizing the eating schedule in order to decrease the risk for abnormal eating episodes (i.e. bingeing or restricting). Bingeing PWDbs are instructed in appropriate timing, quantity, and composition of meals and snacks. The patient must understand why excessively curtailing food (whether it be global or one macronutrient, ie fat, sugar, or carbohydrates) at a particular point or diurnal interval is actually counterproductive and culminates in binge episodes despite an original intent to perpetuate the restriction.

Patients with diabulimia should also be assessed for depression/dysthymia, anxiety, and adjustment disorders, which are shown to have higher incidence rates in Type I. Indeed, any of these are significant etiologies as well as sequelae of juvenile diabetes *and* diabulimia, and sometimes the complex causality is not resolved. We have already discussed how diabulimia is more prevalent in females, and it is likewise of note that Type I females are almost 8 times more likely than males to develop depression post-diagnosis.[26] Patients relate that the cognitive haze induced by chronic or even acute hyperglycemia benumbs sensations of melancholy, desolation, and tedium. (It is unknown as to whether the insulin molecule acts on the brain at a molecular level to provoke depression, or whether the comorbidity can be attributed to the lifestyle changes, behavioral modifications, and normoglycemia that diabetes elicits.) Such practices must be addressed and these appended psychiatric pathologies approached appropriately - it is simple to see how insulin omission to counterbalance feelings of depression can elicit diabulimia, and likewise symptomatologies of anxiety, stress, or maladjustment. If neglected, these concomitant mental illnesses can powerfully inhibit recovery from the insulin-omitting eating disorder. Certain drugs might be administered to effect psychiatric purposes. However, many of these psychotropics also have documented weight gain as a side effect, which is a further likely distressor. (Of note, certain pharmacotherapies are used for the specific treatment of bulimia nervosa, such as selective serotonin reuptake inhibitors, serotonin-norepinephrine reuptake inhibitors, tricyclic antidepressants, and topiramate. These are reported to decrease the cyclical binge/purge cycles inherent to the illness.)

Arguably the most recalcitrant goal facing the mental health professional is to overturn the PWDb's problematic perceptions regarding body image. These are exquisitely layered, intertwined, and difficult to unravel. They thus merit thorough excavation as well as instruction regarding methods of recognition, prevention, and normalization.[30] Addressing this aspect of diabulimia must be a priority, as lingering body dysmorphia 1.) manipulates and derails other positive nuances of the recovery process, 2.) correlates strongly with long-term relapse, and 3.) is validated by contemporary popular culture – rendering correction quite difficult. Approaching self-image perception is generally a segmented process, during which the patient must delve into their own psyche to identify the source of their behaviors. Goal-oriented treatment for this purpose includes 1.) isolating triggers, beliefs, thoughts, and assumptions perpetuating vulnerability to dysmorphia and hindering progress, 2.) eliminating impetuses to compare, contrast, and evaluate self-worth on the basis of body image, 3.) implementing physical and mental techniques to reduce anxiety and stress-related emotions that trigger dysmorphia, 4.) emphasizing "body affirmation" strategies through mirror exposure, engaging in physical activity, and eliminating avoidant behaviors and rituals.[25] It is a long process, and requires dedication and patience from both the patient and psychotherapist (although patients can do so independently).

Perfectionist and obsessive compulsive personality traits are highly comorbid with eating disorders. By promoting fixation on particular entities, these personality traits can trigger disordered eating by generating perceptions of inadequacy and failure. Patients with diabulimia and diabetes, in addition to weight, intake, and shape concerns, are foisted with another avenue of pathological preoccupation – blood sugar levels. Non-diabetic individuals can focus excessively on counting calories and validate themselves through satisfying certain self-imposed limitations or statistics; likewise, a patient with diabetes might develop fastidious control over their glycemic numbers such that aberration from the "normal" perimeters triggers abnormal behaviors in either direction – higher levels of obsession, or complete abandonment (or even periods of both). Perfectionism is associated with most eating disorders and can serve to thwart recovery efforts. The patient might in their own definition 'fail' to manage blood sugar (a cognition/emotion rooted in what they believe to be acceptable, and also their own perceptions of control). On one end of the spectrum, this might lead to greater contraction of dietary or glycemic freedom, opening avenues into other eating pathologies. On the other end, they might become so frustrated or discouraged such that they forego insulin in order to override sensations of futility. (Patients might experience such a profound sense of impotence such that they over-inject themselves in a perilous attempt to regain control, leading to florid hypoglycemia.) Avoiding these avenues necessitates correction of obsessive or perfectionist attitudes towards not only blood sugar but also food and body issues. The clinician should emphasize the benefits of *overall* rather than *micro*-diabetes management, and strike a balance between encouraging conscientiousness as compared to absolute precision. Also, the patient must learn progressively not to blame themselves for wayward blood sugars but rather attribute some such mishaps to extrinsic factors.

Transitioning to different life developmental stages is also facilitated by the mental health professional – namely the individually tailored conversion from prepubescent to adolescent (to young adult to middle age) mindsets. Patients who have undergone a specific type of trauma (here – diagnosis of Type I) or eating disorder (here – diabulimia) manifest characteristics of stunted psychosocial and emotional maturity compared with peers. Due to such illnesses, patients might disengage from their external milieu in favor of internal environments and cognitions, causing them to neglect or abandon normal developmental mores and milestones. The hormonal derangement induced by eating disorders is also an exacerbating factor. Perturbed levels of estrogen/testosterone, growth hormone, parathyroid hormone – not to mention insulin in the case of diabulimia – can all contribute to physical/mental developmental abnormalities. These compounding phenomena are incapacitating during contact with the "real world" again, as induced abruptly by therapy. For example, an adolescent female PWDb might not entirely understand the physical and mental alterations of puberty; likewise, a 20-year-old can misconceptualize her role as a young adult in regards to external attention or expectations. As such, clinicians guide PWDbs through therapy, sensitive to cognitive changes inherent to such intervals.

There are many other aspects to psychotherapy, and are incredibly complex given the circumstantial and historical variations between individual PWDbs. Such miscellanea include factors like family dysfunction – sometimes the core of the patient's disordered behavior lies in perturbations such as divorce, separation, or abuse. Certain family members might attempt to elicit information from the patient to utilize as leverage against another (what is known as triangulation), thereby undermining the concept of a united front. Insulin restriction might be an attempt to draw attention from family members and parents, or regain a margin of control over situations perceived to have gone awry. Some mental health professionals believe that behavioral therapy including the family (if relevant) is absolutely essential for a patient's betterment. Family-based therapy (FBT) has been shown to be efficacious for both anorexia and bulimia nervosa, especially for adolescent and younger patients.[27] Although the dynamics and details of the treatment differ between anorexia and bulimia (namely, the extent of therapist involvement, familial engagement, and patient autonomy), the fundamental principles remain the same. Parents and family members are often encumbered with guilt for the misconception that they 'caused' their child's eating disorder, and as such, this therapy commences with validation and reassurance of parenting skills. The overall (very simplified) individually titrated sequence thereafter involves 1.) dissecting eating patterns by observing meals, 2.) directing parents to institute particular types of eating geared towards weight gain (for anorectic patients) or evasion of cyclical binge-purging (for bulimic patients), 2.) encouraging the family to determine their own mealtime parameters rather than the therapist dictating schedules, for more efficient postprandial monitoring of compliance, 3.) providing a framework for the family to function as a consolidated unit so the patient can amend their eating patterns, and 4.) progressively granting the patient autonomy over their intake after fulfilling therapeutic goals (anorexia – weight gain, bulimia – ceasing binge-purge cycling).

The PWDb's social environment also must be addressed. Seclusion and antisocial behavior can contribute to disordered eating patterns. Isolative practices bolster ritualistic eating, excessive introspection, and physical assessment, all of which diminish the benefits associated with interpersonal interaction. It is much easier for the PWDb to focus on and validate unfavorable thoughts if they remain encloistered, despite conscious recovery efforts in other areas. During therapy, they are encouraged to engage, develop, and/or maintain a comfortable network of people with whom they can productively communicate. The PWDb also nurtures feelings of shame (for inadequacy, lack of control, self-destructive behavior, deceit, and most of all – the 'action' of diabulimia itself) which they prevent themselves from overtly expressing to family and social groups. The patient is prompted to reveal their perceived "skeleton in the closet" to these audiences. This can further help to suppress trepidation or anxiety concerning social interactions.

References:
1.) Fioretto P, Muollo B, Faronato PP, Opocher G., Trevisan R, Tiengo A, Mantero F, Remuzzi G, Crepaldi G, and Nosadini R. "Relationships among Natriuresis, Atrial Natriuretic Peptide and Insulin in Insulin-dependent Diabetes." *Kidney International* 41.4 (1992): 813-21.

2.) Kalambokis, Georgios N., Agathocles A. Tsatsoulis, and Epameinondas V. Tsianos. "The Edematogenic Properties of Insulin." *American Journal of Kidney Diseases* 44.4 (2004): 575-90.

3.) Friedberg, Cylla E., Marjolijn Van Buren, Joost A. Bijlsma, and Hein A. Koomans. "Insulin Increases Sodium Reabsorption in Diluting Segment in Humans: Evidence for Indirect Mediation through Hypokalemia." *Kidney International* 40.2 (1991): 251-56.

4.) Hopkins, D. F., S. J. Cotton, and G. Williams. "Effective Treatment of Insulin-induced Edema Using Ephedrine." *Diabetes Care* 16.7 (1993): 1026-028.

5.) 1.) Ferrannini, E., S. Taddei, D. Santoro, A. Natali, C. Boni, D. Del Chiaro, and D. Buzzigoli. "Independent Stimulation of Glucose Metabolism and Na+-K+ Exchange by Insulin in the Human Forearm." *American Journal of Physiology* 255 (1988).

6.) Nutrition Recommendations and Interventions for Diabetes-2006: A Position Statement of the American Diabetes Association." *Diabetes Care* 29.9 (2008): 2140-157.

7.) Kulkarni, K. D. "Carbohydrate Counting: A Practical Meal-Planning Option for People With Diabetes." *Clinical Diabetes* 23.3 (2005): 120-22.

8.) Knight, E., M. Stampfer, S. Hankinson, D. Speigelman, and G. Curhan. "The Impact of Protein Intake on Renal Function Decline in Women with Normal Renal Function or Mild Renal Insufficiency." *Annals of Internal Medicine* 138 (2003): 460-67.

9.) "The Satiating Power of Protein—a Key to Obesity Prevention." *The American Journal of Clinical Nutrition* 82 (2005)

10.) "Nutrition and Diabulimia Recovery." Telephone interview. 21 July 2011.

11.) Chelliah, Aruna, and Mark R. Burge. "Insulin Edema in the Twenty-first Century: Review of the Existing Literature." *Journal Of Investigative Medicine* 52.02 (2004): 104.

12.) Rozenzweig, JL., Principles of insulin therapy. In: Kahn RC, Weir GC, editors. Joslin's diabetes mellitus. 13th ed. Philadelphia: Lea and Febiger; 1994. p.460-88.

13.) Institute of Medicine: *Dietary Reference Intakes: Energy, Carbohydrate, Fiber, Fat, Fatty acids, Cholesterol, Protein, and Amino Acids.* Washington, DC. National Academic Press. 2002

14.) Saudek, C. D., P. R. Boulter, and R. A. Arky. "The Natriuretic Effect of Glucagon and Its Role in Starvation." *Journal of Clinical Endocrinology & Metabolism* 36.4 (1973): 761-65.

15.) Bent-Hansen, L., B. Feldt-Rasmussen, A. Kverneland, and T. Deckert. "Transcapillary Escape Rate and Relative Metabolic Clearance of Glycated and Non-glycated Albumin in Type 1 (insulin-dependent) Diabetes Mellitus." *Diabetologia* 30.1 (1987): 2-4.

16.) Nestler, J. E., C. O. Barlascini, G. A. Tetrault, M. J. Fratkin, J. N. Clore, and W. G. Blackard. "Increased Transcapillary Escape Rate of Albumin in Nondiabetic Men in Response to Hyperinsulinemia." *Diabetes* 39.10 (1990): 1212-217.

17.) Christlieb, A. R., J. P. Assal, N. Katsilambros, G. H. Williams, G. P. Kozak, and T. Suzuki. "Plasma Renin Activity and Blood Volume in Uncontrolled Diabetes. Ketoacidosis, a State of Secondary Aldosteronism." *Diabetes* 24.2 (1975): 190-93.

18.) Chan ST, Johnson AW, Moore MH, Kapadia CR, Dudley HA. "Early Weight Gain and Glycogen-obligated Water during Nutritional Rehabilitation."*Human Nutrition Clinical Nutrition* 36: 223-32.

19.) Donini, LM, D. Marsili, MP Graziani, M. Imbriale, and C. Canella. "Orthorexia Nervosa: a Preliminary Study with a Proposal for Diagnosis and an Attempt to Measure the Dimension of the Phenomenon." *Eating and Weight Disorders* 9.2 (2004).

20.) Frohnauer, Mary K., James R. Woodworth, and James H. Anderson. "Graphical Human Insulin Time-Activity Profiles Using Standardized Definitions." *Diabetes Technology Therapeutics* 3.3 (2001): 419-29.

21.) Daniel, P.M., E.R. Love, S.R. Moorehouse, O.E. Pratt, and Penelope Wilson. "Factors Influencing Utilisation of Ketone-bodies by Brain in Normal Rats and Rats with Ketoacidosis." *The Lancet* (1971): 637-38.

22.) Goodyear, PhD, Laurie J., and Barbara B. Kahn, MD. "Exercise, Glucose Transport, And Insulin Sensitivity." *Annual Review of Medicine* 49.1 (1998): 235-61.

23.) Marliss, E. B., and M. Vranic. "Intense Exercise Has Unique Effects on Both Insulin Release and Its Roles in Glucoregulation: Implications for Diabetes." *Diabetes* 51.90001 (2002): 271S-83.

24.) Wasserman DH, Lickley HLA, Vranic M: Interactions between glucagon and other counterregulatory hormones during normoglycemic and hypoglycemic exercise. *Journal of Clinical Investigation* 74:1404–1413, 1984.

25.) Cash, Thomas F. *The Body Image Workbook*. New York, NY: MJF, 1997.

26.) Kovacs, M., Goldston, D., Obrosky, D. S., & Bonar, L. K. "Psychiatric disorders in youths with IDDM: Rates and risk factors." *Diabetes Care* (1997): 20, 36–44.

27.) Lock, James, and Daniel LeGrange. *Treatment Manual for Anorexia Nervosa, Second Edition: A Family-Based Approach*. 2nd ed. New York: Guilford, 2013. Web.

28.) Takii, M., Y. Uchigata, G. Komaki, T. Nozaki, H. Kawai, Y. Iwamoto, and C. Kubo. "An Integrated Inpatient Therapy for Type 1 Diabetic Females with Bulimia Nervosa A 3-year Follow-up Study." *Journal of Psychosomatic Research* 55.4 (2003): 349-56.

29.) Katzman, Debra. "Medical Complications in Adolescents with Anorexia Nervosa: A Review of the Literature." *International Journal of Eating Disorders* 37.S1 (2005): 52-59.

30.) Keel, P. K., D. Dorer, D. Franko, S. Jackson, D. Herzog. "Postremission Predictors of Relapse in Women With Eating Disorders."*American Journal of Psychiatry* 162.12 (2005): 2263-268.

CHAPTER 9

RELAPSE

I'm tired of allegory. I wish I didn't have to give you the trite version, because that of course would imply that ours is not unique, that we can be conveniently categorized and shelved to gather dust in the annals of observation. I wish I didn't have to say that he is always lurking in the intimations of shadow, in the subtleties of a floating ribbon, a flash of recollection. He is our parasite, our extortionist, the one who gleefully appropriates every delight and tarnishes them with the rust of apprehension. Where is he now? Are we finally at a stalemate? Or is that him, conspiring in the corner, and I am checkmated yet again?

I live in constant fear of relapse. The dread fades, as the period of diabulimia accrues distance and time, but like the stalker of simile, it traces my every move and lays its pawns in strategic position for the final coup. Did I say final? I apologize – let me qualify. I meant a final that keeps repeating being final. It's an incessant final. Irony's hilarious, isn't it? Every day I have to make sure that my mental defenses are in place, whether this means following a strict regimen of eating, drinking coffee, sleeping, studying, drinking coffee, exercising, and did I mention drinking coffee?

I feel stifled. I feel as if I can't participate in normal activities without meticulous formulations involving time, and calories, and ponderings. I can't go out with friends for an impromptu lunch, or a Friday pizza on movie night, or what if we run late at the bowling alley and everyone votes to get fast food…what must I do then? I wish I could be like them, eat extravagantly and then forget instead of agonizing over each unentitled bite. This is why I avoid such situations as much as possible. The alternative would be relinquishing myself to fate and trusting that my own psychosomatics will subscribe to self-preservation. This would be infinitely easier. You'd think that my own body would fight, tooth and nail, to survive, but it is weak, brittle, vitreous. Treacherous. For who's to say that I won't succumb to leaving out a unit or two of insulin – for a day, a month, then a year. It's inevitable, and every time, it's like developing diabulimia all over again. I'm in a glass labyrinth, and the Minotaur guards the outlet…

Towards Healing

Although the premise of this chapter appears pessimistic, relapse is a core nuance of diabulimia that we cannot overlook. It is a feature common to most eating disorders, but there are key elements which are specific to insulin omission for weight control.

It is important to first define some relevant words so to avoid creating an alphabet soup of terminology. Distinctions between "recovery," "remission," "relapse," and "recurrence" must be made, especially as they relate to subsequent treatment trajectories. In both the vernacular and medical fields, many of these are utilized interchangeably, which confounds cross-institutional standardization as well as public comprehension of the issues. Diabulimia "relapse" is simplistically understood to be a 'return to insulin omission,' when in reality the matter is far more complex. Did the patient actually attain full "recovery" in the first place? To what extent have/are they omitting insulin again – a few units foregone, or failure to dose themselves at all? For how long has the current episode of insulin omission persisted, and likewise for how long prior was there a complete or partial absence of this injurious behavior? What was their baseline level of insulin omission, and is their "relapse" level of omission on par/higher/lower in comparison? Have their eating patterns changed concomitant with the manipulation of insulin dosing? The entire issue is further complicated by lack of concrete criteria defining diabulimia, which unfortunately precludes demarcations of symptomatology. In fact, how to define recovery is an ongoing academic debate in the eating disorder literature at large.

Frank et al. (1991), conceptualized definitions for these terms as an application towards major depressive disorder, which is an illness similar to eating disorders in that they are both neuropsychiatric in origin, and characterized by remissions, relapses, and recoveries.[1] Therefore, some authors have proposed that the qualitative delineations used for depression can also translate to the chronological patterns of disordered eating.[2] Although such stark specificities are rarely used clinically, neither in nomenclature or criteria, they are useful to clarify our usage of the terms. Such minutiae are important nuances of the patient's response to recuperative therapy, and all distinctions are present along the course of diabulimia recovery. [15]

For these definitional purposes, extracting insulin omission from the "inappropriate compensatory behavior" aggregate of typical anorexia and bulimia nervosas (especially given the lack of germane clinical data) is not entirely useful. For simplicity, we can view the issue from the wider perspective of a general eating disorder, and "diabulimia" as a method of execution. However, due to both the 1.) features characteristic of diabetic patients (described later in this chapter) and 2.) sequelae of insulin omission which are not applicable to members of the overall population, insulin omission must also at some points in the discussion be considered a categorical symptom, with "restricting" and "bingeing" subtypes as illustrated in previous chapters.

The *clinical* criteria for "recovery" vary greatly (both inter-institutionally as well as inter-disciplinarily – an endocrinologist might have different interpretations of recovery than a mental health professional), but the purpose of the *theoretical* distinctions here is to provide multiple platforms of analysis. These include namely the 1.) presence/absence (along a spectrum) and relative intensity of symptoms, and 2.) the duration of time

---

[15]   Eating disorders, and especially those involving insulin omission, are interesting in that they also involve characteristics of addiction – namely the psychological and physical dependence on a particular substance, entity, idea, or behavior. In diabulimia, these can be weight loss, diametric extremes of food consumption (bingeing or restricting), the thrill of perceived control, or a combination of the aforementioned – any sequelae of insulin manipulation potentially feeds into attitudes of reliance. The PWDb is not only physically dependent on insulin restriction but also cognitively enslaved to the principle. They live for the next 'euphoria' where low insulin levels gratify both mentally (fulfillment of rapid weight loss, knowledge of caloric purging, transient mollification of dysmorphia), as well as physically (the body readjusts to the hyperglycemia/hypoinsulinemia such that normal glucose and insulin levels leave the patient temporarily unstable). This addiction is twice diabolical with insulin-omitting eating disorders – unlike psychoactive substance/behavioral addiction in the traditional sense, the patient cannot simply attenuate levels of or cease caloric intake /insulin omission 'cold turkey.' *Both* food and insulin are obviously required for existence, and diabetic patients must be especially attentive to their effects throughout the phases of recovery. Their inexorable presence renders extremely difficult the striking of a delicately calibrated balance between awareness and fixation.

for which these symptoms are manifest at such levels. "Observable phenomena" as used here signifies the presence and severity of symptoms or degree of functional status – excluding any incorporation of "duration." The first limits would be "asymptomatic," which, in the case of diabulimia, is the absence of adverse eating behaviors, intentional insulin omission, and other purging behaviors (if initially present). "Fully symptomatic" is defined as a combination of any level of adverse eating behaviors and any amplitude of insulin omission, and "partially symptomatic" signifies what is between.

Duration is the second dimension to incorporate into the definition of these terms. Although explicitly delineated intervals exist in the literature for recovery/remission/relapse/recurrence, they are irrelevant here because 1.) they are used primarily for research purposes - clinicians rarely reference them in practice, electing to use approximations and individually modified criteria, and 2.) these numbers specifically pertain to the overall population and do not incorporate the significantly different mental baselines, etiologies, and purging mechanisms particular to an eating-disordered *diabetic* patient.

Combining observable phenomena with duration yields a clearer illustration of the terms relating to "relapse." A *remission* consists of a minimum period during which the patient is asymptomatic, namely that they are consciously dosing insulin in requisite amounts and adhering to proper daily nutritional and caloric intakes. This remission can be inherently spontaneous; prior treatment is not a contingency. If official treatment is concomitant, however, the psychological member of the diabetic team might attempt cautious tapering of therapy, or at least continue the current regimen.

A *recovery* signifies a *remission* that lasts for greater minimum interval of time. Achieving and maintaining this state is the ultimate goal of eating disorder (and by transitivity - diabulimia – treatment).[16] Further therapy

---

[16] Here, we define 'recovery' by duration as well as the absence of symptoms. However, there are many research-oriented classifications of this nebulous term, and each is swamped in debate. The main parameters of recovery are considered to be nutritional status, menstrual function, mental state, psycho-sexual state, social adjustment, weight (BMI), and bone density. Any of the aforementioned criteria might be used in tandem or in isolation as outcome criteria to evaluate a patient, but this is ultimately the prerogative of the attending physician.

then depends on the discretion and expertise of the physician, who might either elect to terminate treatment, or continue at a less intense grade for the purpose of preventing future return to either partial or full symptomatism.

A *relapse* occurs between these two benchmarks – during the period of remission when the patient is fully/partially asymptomatic, but before the full time to qualify as 'recovered'. It involves a return to full/partial symptomatism of diabulimia – insulin omission of any degree, combined with disordered eating of any type. Contrary to popular understanding, "relapse" does not imply regressing to diabulimia from a fully recovered state. Rather, the patient still harbored mental anomalies during the remission stage which prompted re-expression of purging mechanisms (insulin omission/otherwise) and disordered eating. (Unfortunately, as these measurements rest on the premise of *observable* phenomena, it is not feasible to dissect the likelihood of true recovery from the interim period during which the patient is still susceptible to relapse or recurrence. Physicians can only hypothesize their distinction, given the absence/presence of symptomatic reappearance, and other criteria such as patient function and overall behavior.) As relapse represents a return of the original condition (either full-fledged or partial), it should indicate either the need for a 1.)

One of the most widely used scales in existence today to evaluate the "recovery" of patients with eating disorders was proposed by Morgan and Russell in 1975, which involves a "score" rating of the first five measures mentioned above. Some of these are divided into further assessments: "nutritional status," for example, is an aggregate of 1.) restriction of food intake, 2.) concern about body image, 3.) body weight. "Psychosexual state" is subclassified into 1.) attitude towards sexual matters, 2.) aims in sexual matters, 3.) overt sexual behavior, 4.) attitude towards menstruation if returned or if not returned. "Socioeconomic state" is subclassified into 1.) relationship with family, 2.) emancipation from family, 3.) social contacts outside family, 4.) social activites outside family 5.) employment record. Although physicians rarely assign any patient a "score," these criteria represent useful landmarks of mental improvement. Qualitative – usually not quantitative - use of this system in application to insulin-omitting eating disorders is varied.

Diabulimia is a relatively novel pathology (in recognition, if not in execution) and lacks the requisite breadth and depth of clinical investigations for delineation of remission/recovery criteria. Until experts determine such specifications, clinicians must treat empirically and, ideally, maintain long-term contact with the PWDb to maximize therapeutic permanence.

potent therapeutic intervention if the remission was spontaneous, or 2.) more aggressive course of overall treatment.

Finally, a *recurrence* is similar to a *relapse* in all regards except that it occurs during the period of *recovery*. That is to say, it is a "new" episode, and the patient's chance of experiencing it is no greater than that of the overall population. One of the greatest difficulties – especially concerning such a clinically under-recognized condition as diabulimia – is determining whether a period of diabulimia "recovery" was, in fact, a recovery. Was it actually a prematurely labeled "remission," masquerading as such while the patient still endured concealed cognitive pathology? Assuming that it was, in fact, a true *recovery*, (in which all unfavorable mentation pertaining to weight/eating/shape was abolished), a return to diabulimia symptomatism embodies "recurrence," and thus necessitates recalibration of treatment. The psychological member of the team will consider the reasons for the recurrence, as well as relevant history and course of the patient's illness, in order to most efficiently secure another ('more' indelible) recovery.

The question remains as to exactly the durations of remission and recovery, and how they are differentiated. Although there have been a few cohort studies of eating-disordered diabetic patients practicing insulin restriction at baseline, the time to follow-up and the examinations in the interim were not rigorous enough to determine the intervals detailing these two parameters. The follow-up periods for a majority of these clinical investigations are within the range of 5-10 years, and even if a subject might claim to have amend their eating and insulin adherence, the criteria are quite vague and lack uniformity across studies. Hence, no standard of normalization, let alone quantification, currently exists. (Fortunately, this is not detrimental to the scientists at the helm of such research, as they usually seek to document long-term metabolic complications or overall psychological functioning after *qualitative* omission of insulin for weight control.) Thus, it is currently impractical to pinpoint a precise range for which these variables are legitimate. Physicians and researchers might elect to use an iterative approach towards determining the durations and subsequent treatment approaches for a particular patient, such that each progressive sequence of recovery and/or relapse is modified given the trends noted in the previous cycle.

As we have indicated elsewhere, the particulars of insulin omission especially in light of its highly specific insulin-dependent diabetes demographic, render it far more specialized than conventional purging behaviors. The psychological effects of these singular features – even when considered subordinate to anorexia and bulimia nervosas – are similarly disparate in terms of 1.) the time it takes to effect a remission, 2.) the time necessary for a remission to qualify as a recovery, 3.) how these periods integrate into the definitions for remission and recurrence. To fully dissect these effects, however, we must first describe the myriad factors contributing to recessive behavior in recovering PWDbs (some, but not all of which, overlap with those affecting the non-diabetic eating-disordered population).

Please note that much of the following information has been derived from experiences with and narratives from patients and physicians – it is difficult to issue consensus statements from the literature as few studies have had the longitudinal opportunity to statistically validate such qualitative observations.

Intra-treatment Pre-remission

The period *after* treatment initiation and *prior* to fulfillment of remission criteria is essentially when the PWDb is most vulnerable to recessive behavior. Many nefarious factors present in synchrony to dissuade the patient from their amenability to therapy, and these continue to operate indefinitely – infiltrating even remission and recovery phases. During this period, the most nebulous (albeit highly potent) devil is the tantalizingly proximal "reminiscence" of diabulimia. When besieged on all fronts by edema, hunger, despondence, insulin refraction, and many other anti-recovery dynamics, the PWDb often has nothing to look back upon save the period of diabulimia itself, which begins to appear incredibly appetizing again. There is no "Look how far I've come," no precedent of success, no source of positive reinforcement restraining them from another (or primary) relapse into insulin omission. No – oftentimes the only sinister consolation derives from a retrospectively-biased memory of the convenience of life with diabulimia, the ease of keeping the weight off without even really trying, the satisfaction of freedom to eat anything whenever and wherever. If not for any other reason than that insulin omission is still "fresh in the mind," surviving this initial phase is no paltry feat, and represents one of the toughest triumphs over the illness.

In regards to multidisciplinary treatment with a diabetic team (as opposed to self-medication), this pre-remission interval includes a dangerous "Siberia" of sorts. Official psychotherapy cannot begin unless the patient's blood sugars are marginally normalized, as hyperglycemia reversibly disturbs neural circuitry and leaves the patient unfocused, confused, and suboptimally functional. Until such glycemic levels are achieved, the patient undergoes a more educational approach to well-being rather than active treatment. This period, during which the patient is expected to correct physiology without simultaneous mental redress, leaves them perilously vulnerable to dynamics inducing diabulimia in the first place. Tragically, much resolve towards improvement wanes or is even wholly relinquished in these first few days (or weeks, or months – however long glycemic repair requires. See Chapter 8: Treatment.)

Edema is also one of the most potent adversaries. As described in the previous chapter, the rapid 10-30 pound fluid appendage following insulin treatment (leaving many patients heavier than they were prior to beginning insulin omission) is devastating. It prompts reevaluation of rationale for treatment compliance, and many (especially PWDbs who have undergone multiple cycles of remission and relapse) know that eliminating insulin again can overturn the acute increase in weight. In the words of one patient, "I've been through recovery and relapse so many times that I can't even count…no matter how many times I cycle, edema is the one thing that frightens me the most. Even though I know it goes away, how do I tell myself that? How do you block the million questions and doubts popping up in your head?…*Maybe that's not just water, maybe what I ate last night is making me fat…That one time I gave myself insulin for that binge – maybe that means this isn't going to go away… Why is it taking so long – is this part actually permanent?*…and it freaks me out more than you can imagine…"

However, all weight gain is not necessarily a spontaneously reversible fluid retention. Insulin is the quintessential anabolic hormone, and patients who dose themselves correctly might indeed experience a physiological upsurge in fat and carbohydrate storage. Indeed, studies have shown body mass increases in patients undergoing aggressive insulin therapy even in the absence of caloric excess.[4] This compounding of weight gain and apparent irreversibility similarly antagonize the patient's desire to defeat diabulimia, prompting both acute and long-term return to disordered behaviors. Weighing machines are as such contraindicated during the initial stages of treatment prior to edema resolution – if the PWDb is provided numerical substantiation of increasing body mass in addition to the physical manifestations of swelling and perceptible tightness in the extremities, significant distress and potential relapse can ensue.

Another anti-recovery process presenting during the pre-remission stage is temporary 'unresponsiveness' to insulin and consequent frustration with unpredictable glucose values. Striated tissues are temporarily desensitized to the hormone after extended hyperglycemia (secondary to downregulation of the cell surface insulin receptor), such that a greater dose is required to incur the same effect on blood sugar. The renal insulin clearance is also uncharacteristically heightened during this period, yielding both less insulin and a shorter period of time for tissue employment. Perceptions of futility, vexation, demoralization, concern, anger, perplexity, and inadequacy may result from refractory blood glucose readings, leaving the PWDb more vulnerable to relapse. (Many patients with eating disorders exhibit perfectionist traits, which only serves to exacerbate the problem as relatively smaller deviations will launch the same magnitude of reactive capacity.) Like edema and appetite, insulin refraction eventually recedes – but this also creates a problem in the form of hypoglycemia. The return to appropriate insulin response is neither abrupt nor predictable and the patient might experience hypoglycemic excursions secondary to an excess of insulin which would originally have qualified as an appropriate dose. Hypoglycemia, in addition to catalyzing binge episodes, likewise can lead to incompetence, frustration, and erroneous internal attributions, all of which are ingressions into relapse.

Heightened appetite following reinstitution of insulin is more common with bingeing PWDbs (not typically the restrictive subtype, as they have already acclimatized to the physical promptings of caloric shortage). Bingeing PWDbs who use excessive caloric restriction as a purging mechanism (in addition to insulin omission) may be especially susceptible to appetite increase, as they might intentionally undereat to control weight in the presence of normoinsulinemia. (Hyperglycemia/hypoinsulinemia also induces pathologic hunger, but in this situation bingeing PWDbs are permitted satiation knowing that the excess calories will not "stick.") Insulin even under normal circumstances activates molecular hunger cascades, and its more conspicuous presence in the bloodstream during diabulimia treatment powerfully increases the somatic and often unjustifiable provocation to consume calories. A patient recuperating from an eating disorder might take unfavorably to these visceral promptings. In response to hunger, the PWDb can either 1.) yield to compulsion or 2.) restrain themselves. The former results in concern over further weight gain, which if permitted accruement over time will prompt compensatory behaviors – insulin omission or otherwise. Both reactions can lead to binge episodes if the PWDb has not yet learned through psychotherapy how to stifle these occurrences. And bingeing, as has been underscored, almost inexorably incurs insulin omission especially in a patient already familiar with the 'benefits' of such action. Even if the PWDb doses themselves for the binge episode despite concern over the effects of excess consumption, the consequent sensation of failure may be detrimental to overall therapeutic compliance. The insulin/normoglycemia-induced hunger eventually tapers as the body acclimatizes to a new nutritional baseline, but is a difficult milestone to overcome in the acute phases of treatment.

Nutrition itself can contribute towards relapse during this inter-treatment pre-remission gap, especially in light of the insulin and appetite dyscrasias outlined above. All of the factors discussed in the previous chapter (e.g., macronutritional and caloric recommendations) exacerbate the elaborate knowledge that the eating-disordered diabetic patient often possesses. The technological upsurge in the past decade has lent the insulin-dependent diabetic greater flexibility concerning the types of food ingested, but patients still harbor the misconception that certain foods are "anti-diabetic" or "anti-weight control." The PWDb can progress to symptoms of depression given the apprehension accompanying the loss of caloric freedom they held during insulin omission. (Even returning to a totally normal caloric consumption may feel like severe restriction for a previously bingeing PWDb, who is somatically and psychologically accustomed to greater intake levels.) *True* caloric/macronutritional restriction, on the other hand, is toxic especially to a patient manifesting an aberrant mental baseline. These extended periods of caloric/macronutritional abstinence lead to insidious upregulation and accumulation of 1.) molecular and 2.) psychological signals promoting consumption of the food(s) under limitation, both of which erupt given the proper propellant ('abstinence-violation' effect).

In a nefarious psychological cycle, relapse itself can lead to relapse – especially in this preliminary period. Omitting even *one* qualitative dose provides any combination of the following: 1.) powerfully rapid positive reinforcement of body mass control with water weight loss, 2.) feelings of failure, fear, and frustration, which strengthen the idea that recuperation is unrealistic, 3.) sensations of liberation and relief from worrying about metabolizing 'illicit' calories, 4.) impetus to omit 'just one more dose,' which of course leads to indefinite perpetuation. These seeds are implanted deeper into the patient's mind, and render future attempts at recovery proportionally harder.

There is currently no consensus favoring either the insulin pump or injections as risk factors for relapse. Although both modalities have their advantages and disadvantages, neither one has definitively been shown to confer benefit or harm over the other.

Relapse

After the patient achieves remission, many of the acute factors described above (in addition to qualitatively novel types of attacks) persist in their potential to impel relapse. Stated crudely, the world is immediately and longitudinally anti-recovery. Precipitating antecedents like hunger, edema, subpar glycemic and HbA1c values, and objectively/subjectively inappropriate caloric intake might flare in particular daily circumstances, even after the patient has persevered for a certain length of time adhering to appropriate eating and insulin patterns. (Fortunately, these are somewhat weakened as compared to the pre-remission stage.) Acute hunger attacks can derive randomly or through improper eating schedules. Likewise, edema might persist indefinitely or reappear following an isolated high glucose value. Hyper/hypoglycemia is generally manageable, but extenuating circumstances are sometimes involved in recalcitrant glucose levels, and not all are expressly provoked by the PWDb's actions.

Recall here that 'relapse' is a return to symptomatic behavior in a period of remission, compared to "recurrence," which is symptomatism in a period of recovery. A reversion to purging can involve insulin omission, vomiting/laxatives/diuretics, excessive exercise, or any combination of the above. Note that a patient can return to conventional purging behaviors *without* insulin omission, or vice versa, or both. (Non-insulin-omitting disordered eating/purging can nevertheless culminate in insulin restriction). Similarly, eating patterns can entail either restricting and/or bingeing. Prior consumption habits, such as those present in the initial episode of diabulimia or during past relapses, do not necessarily dictate those manifest during the current relapse. (They are, however, more likely to be predictive.) An interesting study of eating disordered patients without diabetes noted that previously anorexic patients were more likely during relapse to cross over to bulimic/bingeing behaviors rather than vice versa, perhaps validating the theory of physiological recompense from periodic starvation.[6]

Factors contributing to relapse may be *qualitatively* similar to those experienced by any non-diabetic eating-disordered remissive patient, if not entirely *quantitatively: identities* of relapse stimulants are comparable between the two groups, but their magnitude and duration often are not. As detailed, the conscientious diabetic patient's baseline awareness of nutrition and calories is often, and requisitely, elevated as compared to their non-diabetic peers. Diabetes yields their threshold for eating pathology much lower as a population. The etiologies underlying such conditions can similarly galvanize relapse, and require slighter triggers for a shorter periods to provoke the same inappropriate action. It is proportionally harder for a diabetic patient to see/eat food and not dwell upon it (for whatever reason – carbohydrates and insulin dosing are the most common, but portion size, sugars, calories, and fat might soon follow) than it is for an non-diabetic individual.

Imagery, especially that from the media, can also propel flares of distorted behavior. Media and marketing promote both overt and subliminal messages perpetuating the need to attain an 'ideal' body.

External environments are replete with affirming depiction of individuals with low weight, high fitness, and muscularity. Tragically, these are selected from few and broadcasted to many, endorsing a false 'reality.' This surplus can function to advantage and/o r detriment, as 1.) completely ineffectual or 2) a positive source of motivation to be healthier/lose weight/develop strength, etc.

In a remissive eating-disordered patient, however, these factors are prone to psychological magnification. Termed 'media internalization' this promotes certain superlatives perceived as either 'be-all-end-all,' or completely inaccessible. Images undeniably intermesh with the patient's appraisal of their own body, which is generally tied to the values substantiated by their surroundings. Mirrors, weighing machines, measuring tapes, clothes – all serve to consolidate body dysmorphia. These misconceptions can derive from a particular body part or feature (such as the flatness of the stomach or the curvature of the nose), or the body as a whole (such as size or silhouette). They are subsequently bolstered through comparison with 1.) external influences persuaded by the information, imagery, and opinion present in the environment (for example, comparison to an apparently 'more attractive' peer), or 2.) internally encoded ideals (for example, the restrictive PWDb who strives for lower weight despite far surpassing the social perimeters of 'thin'). If psychotherapy does not adequately train to nullify these mentations, the restrictive *or* bingeing PWDb might again seek out abnormal behaviors. These distorted impressions are unique to neither the remission nor pre-eating disorder periods, and reappear in greater potency and titer unless the patient takes measures towards their inhibition.

In a related note, weight gain is also a common source of relapse. Metabolic (not fluid) weight gain *after* the initial insulin edema phase can be acute or gradual (although the process is more frequently insidious than it is overt). Some time is necessary for the patient to readjust to the lower caloric intake demanded by normoinsulinemia, and the now assimilated caloric excess leads to chronic tissue deposition. Bingeing episodes, on the other hand (as are sometimes present even in the remission period), not only provide an acute caloric overload, but also concomitant water retention. The combination of true-mass and fluid weight gain engenders panic, anxiety, and consternation sourcing from future transgressions.

Accidental hyperglycemia for whatever reason also causes temporary edema after correction, which might be perceived as a sudden and unjustifiable increase in mass. Edema for these *acute* excursions of hyperglycemia-to-normoglycemia are usually relatively less prolonged than those following chronic insulin-deficient intervals (but these intervals are patient-specific).

Verbal provocations are also common and important to consider. Most salient are comments concerning weight, which can be inadvertent or intentional in their reference. Comments such as "You've gained weight," or "Are you sure you want to eat that?" should undeniably be avoided, but even phrases that to the normal ear sound completely harmless (or even flattering) can be perceived as offensive to the remissive PWDb, e.g. "You look much healthier," or "You've filled out nicely." These sentences, which in most circumstances are intended graciously, can be cognitively construed as "Oh, they must mean I've gotten fat," "How bad did I look before?" or "'Healthy' is a euphemism for 'fat.'" In some cases, 'normality' is a concept expressly shunned by the PWDb, and implying (through these types of apparently laudatory remarks) that they belong in this category intimates a loss of control, singularity, or exclusivity.

Patients deeply internalize the opinions and remarks of their families, friends, and colleagues according to their own (and often problematic) interpretations and associations. For example, issuing offhand remarks as those aforementioned (or any to similar effect) is essentially analogous to handing a foaming beer to a recovering alcoholic. It brings to working memory those sensations of imperfection, deficit, shame, and frustration, which quietly reseed the mind and feed parasitically on anything else that reinforces their toehold. The toehold becomes a foothold, a stronghold – ad infinitum – profoundly perturbing the patient's remissive equanimity and leading to old behaviors.

Another verbal instigator involves encouraging the PWDb to eat more – an incitation inspired perhaps by observing the patient's weight or consumption patterns. Throughout all phases of treatment/recovery, the PWDb can maintain very disciplined eating regimens – this is due to a combination of 1.) healthy diabetes management and 2.) positive effort towards weight and appetite control. Alternatively, this cultivated discipline might border on pathological, favoring perhaps excessively restricted intake.

The remissive PWDb generally does not appreciate coercion (inadvertent or otherwise) to stray from this imposed routine – they understand their own vulnerabilities concerning food and have attempted to institute appropriate defenses. Coaxing greater intake, while conceivably justified, is immediately and profoundly destabilizing.

By the same token, dissuading the PWDb from eating can also prove dangerous. This can stem from the [parent/friend/colleague]'s concern about diabetes management, which serves only to reinforce the myth that the diabetic is fettered by default from conventional pleasures such as eating what everyone else can eat. Discouraging caloric intake can also be prompted by judgment regarding the patient's weight. The latter only reinforces the PWDbs baseline dysmorphia.

Aspects of food and eating themselves, at face value, can elicit regressive behavior. They are a ubiquitous part of daily existence, and patients obviously cannot completely eliminate them from consciousness during remission and recovery periods. Relapse can be precipitated by a plethora of food-related permutations: the 'memory' of diabulimia and its convenient eradication of intake consequences, the consciousness of food and its limitations/effects, the metabolic impetus to eat after intentional but non-pathological constraint, ingestion of a food deemed by the PWDb to be inappropriate, excessive caloric and portion and macronutrient quantification, and appetite itself.

Similar to that of the body, depiction of food is abundant within the public sphere via internet, magazines, stores, restaurants. Its portrayal as a superlative source of pleasure, voluminous audiovisual products in their gory and saliva-inducing detail, illustrations of gratuitous customer enjoyment – all are simultaneously vilified and glorified as 'food pornography' given the apparently innocuous yet explicit nature of their presentations. These images actually have a physiological basis in that the simple thought of food/eating (termed the 'cephalic' phase of digestion), releases gastric juices, promotes salivation, and increases gastric motility, all contributing to physical and psychological intensification of appetite. The militant self-control that patients with anorexia, bulimia, and EDNOS impose upon themselves is sometimes derived from the necessity to curtail caloric consumption in the midst of these frenetic images, writings, and advertisements relating to *both* food and body image. Look to the right (often literally), and the slim, beautiful model or sinewy athlete is lionized; look to the left, and a sumptuous cheeseburger lasciviously mocks in its 10x-lifesize billboard magnificence. For a PWDb already sensitized to food and weight and blood sugar and insulin, the situation consummately translates to the vernacular 'between a rock and a hard place,' and 'wanting to have the cake and eat it, too.' While other factors certainly contribute towards the development of disordered eating or the instigation of relapse, such circumstances make it thrice easier to either indulge/binge, or – polarically – deny the existence of food.

Failure of adherence to one therapeutic constituent – whether it is proper nutrition or glucose control – can destabilize and infiltrate into all treatment compartments. For example, take a patient who manages their blood sugars but cannot amend their eating habits. They might consequently view the failure of one management component to preclude total malfunction or render useless the productivity of the others, such that all efforts are foregone. This has clear implications for the balance/velocity of holistic treatment.

The presence of post-diabulimia medical complications can also factor into relapse. One salient influence for complying with treatment is to regain health and equanimity, but the patient has little to no therapeutic reinforcement given the perseverant damage resulting from extended hyperglycemia. The often irreversible somatic sequelae of diabulimia are not only psychologically wearisome but can also physically incapacitate the patient. Peripheral neuropathy is terribly painful, gastroparesis stimulates severe nausea and vomiting, retinopathy produces compromised vision and in some cases permanent blindness, kidney damage protracts the orthoinsulinemic edema, and the list continues. Fatalist attitudes detrimental to maintained compliance ensue, as well as depressive symptoms and sensations of futility.

A baseline decline in psychosocial functioning is another ramification of eating disorders themselves, especially diabulimia. This is attributed not only to cognitive disturbances, but also to physical derangements sourcing from malnutrition and protracted hyperglycemia (including demyelination, metabolite accumulation, rearrangement of neural circuitry, among others). Such changes are largely irreversible, and contribute to worsened (or progressively worsening) social skills and distorted self-perception. Insulin habits and dietary practices specific to diabetes intrinsically galvanize sensations of nonconformity and shame, leading the PWDb to isolate themselves or restrict social engagement to conceal this part of their existence. If these processes are allowed progression, the patient becomes uncomfortable with interpersonal interactions and compensates through seclusion. Seclusion, in turn, is a ripe environment for fixation on cognitions and introspection that can lead ultimately to relapse.

Recapitulating the discussion thus far projects an impression that relapses derive from psychologically 'negative' cognitions, attitudes, results, or sensations. While valid in a majority of cases, this assessment undercuts the incidence of relapse secondary to psychologically 'positive' feelings or occurrences. The practices of insulin omission and other purging behaviors are unique in that some argue that they resemble "addictive" behavior – to weight loss, control, negation of eating, etc. Greater 'doses' are progressively necessary to elicit the same mental effect, and treatment involves ablation or attenuation of the adverse behavior. As such, abstinence from these 'drugs' – while remaining the therapeutic goal, can also inspire entitlement for 'reward,' namely, engaging in prior behavior while in a period of defined remission. The "I've been good, I deserve a drink" attitude is actually extremely perilous, and represents a fiendish cognitive curveball that at face value is not perceived as such. Token for token, these thoughts can be more difficult to resist than relapse triggers derived from 'negative' circumstances, secondary to their apparent innocuity. The PWDb's incentive for seeking reward through insulin omission can be intermeshed with 1.) positive progress in diabulimia therapy, 2.) independently positive circumstances (e.g. commemorative events, finding a job, receiving a good grade, losing weight, having a healthy baby), or 3.) synergistic combination of both. This begins with the overtly harmless consideration of "Oh, it'll be okay this once... I've done well – I want to/should celebrate." The patient proceeds to restrict insulin for what they promise themselves will only be a short entitled period, but of course the original intention is rarely honored. One insulin injection becomes two, two becomes a day's worth, a day – a week, *ad infinitum*. Gratification received from one short breach is only highlighted by the immediately preceding normoinsulinemic period of what the patient might yet consider 'deprivation' from the 'drug' of diabulimia. Creating a fresh cycle of positive reinforcement leads to consequential dread of return to propriety, which by default entails elimination of the drug/reward. This is an important concept – an intentional 'once' is usually never an actual 'once' in the reality of relapse. Frequently the patient must or will run the gamut of another extended diabulimia episode (days to years) before they become acquiescent to therapy once again.

We also do not wish to imply that relapses are entirely psychosomatic in provenance. They can sometimes derive from purely goal-oriented and *premeditated* cognitions related to weight, eating, or singular circumstances. Consider the following:

1.) 'I want to lose 10 pounds before I wear my swimsuit, so I'm going to…'
2.) 'I don't want this calorie-laden meal to stick to my hips, so I'm going to...'
3.) 'I want to get my parents' attention, so I'm going to...'
...*skip my shot today or for the next few days UNTIL I have accomplished this.*

These represent completely intentional ingressions into previous behavior, and are only abetted by the immediate physical convenience (never mind long-term vexations) of insulin omission. (Of note, these same cognitions might also underlie the initial episode of diabulimia.) And, as described above, once is never once – the patient-predetermined limit does little to curtail the harmful behaviors once they are set in motion. Diabulimia again lends its intoxicating perception of control, and the patient is drawn deeper into the jaws of relapse.

This list is absolutely not comprehensive. Relapse is exquisitely complex in its etiology, and it would be impossible to describe the variations intrinsic to each patient. Many of the above, however, are common either in isolation or in combination. Indeed, very often many have symbiotic relationships and their interaction produces potentiating effects on relapse. As such, any of these weaknesses should be addressed during multidisciplinary treatment in as full a capacity and with as much sensitivity as warranted.

<u>Recurrence</u>

We have taken 'recurrence' as a return to symptomatic behavior after an extended period of time sans observable manifestations (aka 'recovery'). Namely, it is a completely new episode without carryover from the previous eating disorder, and essentially implies that the individual was no more likely to have developed it than a member of the general population (diabetic or non-diabetic). As mentioned prior, the following observations have not been empirically validated, and are summarized from patient/clinician testament.

Mechanisms contributing to recurrence are similar to those of relapse. Trigger identities are typically indistinguishable, but their magnitudes and durations are often increased. For example, take a patient whose pathology is induced by deviant blood sugar levels. During *remission*, a relapse into insulin omission or purging behaviors might require one or a few of these occurrences. On the other hand, during *recovery*, many more (qualitatively) abnormal glucose readings for a protracted period of time might be necessary in order to elicit the same behaviors. (This is not to say that identical precipitants act in the same patient across relapse/recurrences – many in fact learn through psychotherapy or self-treatment to pinpoint, suppress, and defeat specific activators, only to have completely unanticipated volleys from left field.)

We have thus far largely bypassed the overlap between diabetic and non-diabetic provocations for the sake of diabulimia specificity. These similar factors adopt greater significance during recurrence. This is attributed to the PWDb's greater psychological normalization towards that of the non-diabetic population. For example, bingeing/restrictive eating and perturbations in recovery maintenance are frequently brought about by both subtle and drastic alterations in circumstances, environment, and occupation – none of which are necessarily diabetes-specific. Similar to the diagnosis of diabetes, which provides a potent source of trauma contributing to the development of disordered eating, some stressful events (e.g. loss of employment, death of a relative/friend, diagnosis of significant illness, and major relocation) are all poisonous to the recovered diabulimia psyche.

Epidemiological studies have demonstrated that the length of the recovery period correlates with the incidence of recurrence. Patients who maintained asymptomatic behavior for relatively longer periods had lower rates of completely new disordered-eating episodes. During this extended period, the patient will have the opportunity to accrue mental normalization and techniques with which to abolish deviant cognitions. It is true that acutely stressful events are often unpredictable and more likely to lead to immediate recurrence; however, the PWDb over years will have learned to 'anticipate the unanticipated' and institute appropriate defenses. The longer this interval, the more resilient the psyche, and the greater the advantage. The disturbance can thereby be thwarted, or require a heftier dose to inspire the same reaction.

As a note to family and healthcare providers – presence of remissive periods during which the PWDb appears to attend to their diabetes regimen *does not preclude* a successive instance of the disorder. Many families who know that their relative has 'recovered' thenceforth ignore any misgiving of diabulimia simply because it is 'in the past,' or attribute the 'same old' symptoms to another more benign etiology. This is a dangerous problem both in the short-term (patients in remission for a few weeks to months) as well as long-term. It is most important to consider in a patient manifesting extended periods of asymptomatism, as observers assume that this negates the *de novo* appearance of suspicious signs. As is true with other eating disorders, protracted vigilance is unfortunately necessary for any diabetic patient with a previous history of diabulimia.

Learning to avoid relapse and recurrence may be profoundly dependent upon psychotherapy. For patients unable to afford or refusing to accept clinical treatment, such processes can be self-taught or conceptualized, but the methods are independent of the elected treatment medium. (Official psychotherapy does, however, lend more structure, guidance, titration, and momentum for maintenance. Often, extended communication with a mental health professional is obligate for years after remission/recovery is attained.) Cognitive or behavioral approaches might be adopted, but treatment for diabulimia is a tailored combination of both. Although this component follows directly from and overlaps with the type of therapy that the patient receives during the initial phases of diabulimia therapy, it is distinct in that it is geared more towards prevention rather than elimination.

The first principle inculcated is trigger recognition. This involves retrospective and prospective identification of weaknesses – both external and internal – that the patient still harbors. They are challenged to understand why these particular entities can spark distorted thinking and adverse emotional responses. Once the beliefs underlying such provocations are extracted, patients can learn to gradually overturn them. Defenses are implemented to weaken or blunt their intrusions, such that they are rendered successively impotent in their attacks. Take, for example, a PWDb in remission who happens upon a intentionally self-restricted food. Problematic mentation can include: "I'm too overweight to eat that," "Eating that will make me fat," and/or "I'm not allowed to have so many carbohydrates/fats/calories." Likewise, another patient might look at a deviant blood glucose reading with "I'm such a failure," "I'm not capable of managing my diabetes," "Why even try when clearly my efforts are to no avail?" The therapist and patient together (or patient independently) go to the source of these distortions and attempt to systematically derail and incapacitate them.

Apparent 'failure' of therapy itself is also addressed – a patient who experiences an acute or extended relapse into insulin omission might think "I've lost all control," "This is great – why did I ever decide to get back on insulin?" and/or "Therapy clearly is not helping." Addressing this nuance is crucial, because short periods of regressive behavior during diabulimia treatment/remittance are common and must not be construed as failure. No matter how trivial, such thinking might chronically or even permanently subvert recovery processes.

Behavioral approaches include 'desensitization' – through gradual exposure to, as well as concentrated abstinence from, the reaction towards environmental or intrinsic triggers. "Starting low and going slow" helps the patient systematically accustom themselves to these mental assaults in incrementally larger doses, until they can be confronted in full potency with minimal evidence of adverse responses. A singular (albeit controversial) approach of some rehabilitation center includes having the patient learn gradually to eat at unfamiliar venues without knowing the food's caloric or macronutrient content, in order to suppress quantification fears, eliminate 'avoidant' eating behaviors, and slowly reintroduce them to proper food approaches. However, until this can be undertaken in a controlled setting under therapist supervision, the PWDb is discouraged from tackling such vulnerabilities. (As such, the self-treating patient is faced with a 'catch-22' in that they must either permanently avoid such susceptibilities, or strongly risk relapse by progressive exposure.)

Some of these factors, however, cannot be rectified and avoidant behavior must be instituted. This involves bypassing what the PWDb, and most normal people, would seek to avoid in the first place. Abusive/destructive relationships – possibly with family, colleagues, and/or significant others, and substance addictive behavior (alcohol, recreational drugs, medications) are obviously malignant. Preoccupation on recipes, preparation, and handling of food (while a more subtle peril) should be limited to that required for existence and no further, as it is difficult for the PWDb to determine what level of fixation is marginally dangerous. Similar principles apply to numerical quantification of the body (measuring and weighing should be minimized to 'spot' appraisals and not referenced for chronological changes in body mass or shape), wearing or modeling particular articles of clothing that highlight imperfections, and engaging in situations which can capitalize on the patient's perceived shortcomings.

References:
1.) Frank, E., R. Prien, R. Jarrett, M. Keller, D. Kupfer, P. Lavori, J. Rush, and M. Weissman. "Conceptualization and Rationale for Consensus Definitions of Terms in Major Depressive Disorder." *Archives of General Psychiatry* 48 (1991).

2.) Field, A., D. Herzog, M. Keller, J. West, K. Nussbaum, and G. Colditz. "Distinguishing Recovery from Remission in a Cohort of Bulimic Women: How Should Asymptomatic Periods Be Described?" *Journal of Clinical Epidemiology* 50 (1997): 1339-345.

3.) Mitchell, J., L. Davis, and G. Goff. "The Process of Relapse in Patients with Bulimia."*International Journal of Eating Disorders* 4 (1985): 457-63. Print.

4.) Purnell, J., J. Hokanson, S. Marcovina, M. Steffes, P. Cleary, and J. Brunzell. "Effect of Excessive Weight Gain With Intensive Therapy of Type 1 Diabetes on Lipid Levels and Blood Pressure." *Journal of the American Medical Association* 280.2 (1998): 140-46.

5.) Herzog DB, Dorer DJ, Keel PK, Selwyn SE, Ekeblad ER, Flores AT, Greenwood DN, Burwell RA, Keller MB. "Recovery and relapse in anorexia and bulimia nervosa: a 7.5-year follow-up study." *J Am Acad Child Adolesc Psychiatry* (1999): 38:829–837

6.) Keel, P. K., D. Dorer, D. Franko, S. Jackson, D. Herzog. "Postremission Predictors of Relapse in Women With Eating Disorders."*American Journal of*

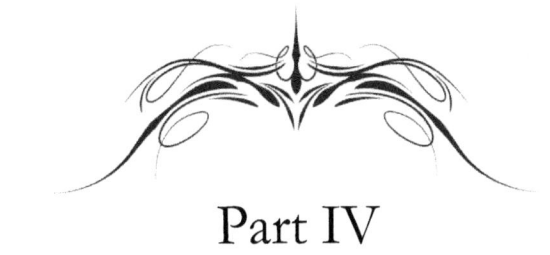

Part IV

APPENDICES

CHAPTER 10

LIVING WITH DIABULIMIA:

FIELD NARRATIVES

Towards Healing

The following narratives are, although holistically fictional, compiled with creative license from the real experiences of patients and relatives of patients suffering from diabulimia. They are included for the intention of illustrating from first-person perspectives the daily travails of those whom this illness touches. Different clues are interspersed to illustrate the concepts presented in the Screening and Execution chapters.

Becky, age 17

Where should I start? Not just chronologically, but symptomatically...Diabulimia is a carnival of satire – one time, one attitude can lend you a delusion of utter invincibility, another day relinquishes you to the floor in lethargic uselessness, others in pounding panic or throes of despair or serenely calm rationalization. I can philosophize the day away, but that's not going to illustrate much. So I'll begin during a forgettable afternoon, when diabulimia was suitably muzzled and tied to a post in the corner of the room.

My classmates and I were all sitting in the dungeon of English class – my senior year of high school we were forced to listen to the drone of Mr. Taylor's voice describing the principle of iambic pentameter, and I *really, really* needed to use the bathroom. The seconds ticked by on the austere clock above the wall, each minute seeming to herald a further expansion of my already-full bladder. *Come on, seriously*...I prayed, hoping that I would be able to hold it in after the bell rang, when I would have to sprint halfway across the school to finally relieve myself. Then the whole cycle would begin again, and after two periods I would have to relive the same torture again. I'd gotten pretty skilled at it, though – I'd figured out a few good staccato breathing techniques and particular sitting positions to make myself a little less uncomfortable. I honestly didn't even notice anymore, that I had to pee every two hours or less.

My friends sometimes wondered, though. One of them even followed me into the bathroom a few times, to make sure I wasn't vomiting or something. It wasn't any secret that I was pretty thin, and to others that fact was probably compounded by virtue of the volume of food I was able to scarf down. I think I ate more calories than the totality of my group of friends combined, to the amazement of anybody who watched me. I'd buy the unhealthiest things I could find, the junk with the highest ratios of sugar and fat. I was even capable of finishing my friends' leftovers after my tray was polished. "I'm such a bad diabetic," I would josh around with everyone, to allay any suspicion. Not as if they would have known anything about what I was doing.

I didn't eat that much entirely on purpose. I *was* insatiably and forever hungry. Even if I didn't take my insulin and tried not to eat, I couldn't do it – it was excruciatingly difficult. Sure, I knew that having high blood sugar entailed that ravenous appetite, but I couldn't seem to cultivate the discipline to fight the hunger. I was keeping the weight off anyway, so something must have been working. On top of that, if I could eat tasty things that everyone had to avoid for the vague purpose of health, who was arguing? Certainly not me.

That day's canteen menu consisted of mozzarella sticks and curly fries, with some questionable red velvet cake for dessert. Mom had packed two peanut butter sandwiches with carrot sticks, but I bought the cafeteria food anyway and inhaled everything, saving the Twinkie for snack in physics class. I made sure to stop at the drinking fountain to fill my industrial-sized water bottle before rushing off to the bathroom and then to 6th period. Today was lab, so I didn't have time to drink anything until my mouth became so parched that I could barely croak out Kepler's second law to my partner. The thirst was manageable, I gulped down half a liter and went back to fiddling with equations without much contemplation. At the end of class our professor put the answers to the lab on the overhead projector so that we could check our work. Normally I was able to discern the fine print from my seat in the back third of the room, but somehow everything was strangely blurry. *Huh.* Maybe I need to switch my contact lenses, two weeks might already have passed.

The remainder of the day was pretty uneventful – I desperately tried to do my calculus problem set in study hall, but my eyelids were so heavily weighted that I had to indulge myself one micronap. *Indulge myself, hah.* I don't think it qualifies as an indulgence if it happens every day...hell, its not just study hall. I drowse off in nearly every class...the only thing keeping me awake is my obnoxious bladder. Mr. Winslow yelled at me once – probably felt insulted that this might be a reflection that none of his lectures were worth staying awake for – but I just joked with him that I seemed to be suffering from bouts of narcolepsy and he let me off the hook. Lately, I've been cultivating the skill of sleeping with my eyes open – if only my eyelids would follow suit by staying suspended. It's a work in progress.

"400's today! You ready?" Jen called across the hall lockers at me as we packed up for track practice after tenth period. My books were so heavy...when did my physics text start to weigh 15 pounds.

"Ah, blast, 400's?" I groaned and heaved my backpack onto my shoulders, securing the straps firmly across my waist, tightening them slightly. "I think I might just dog them today. Who ever has energy for 400's? You're totally insane for sounding this excited."

She looked marginally irritated. "You're always dogging practice these days. Even the 800s. What's up with you?" She grabbed one of the looser straps of my pack and yanked it across my narrow chest. "You always look like you've just been stun-gunned. Not sick, are you?"

"Don't think so. No fever, I'll be okay I guess. Senioritis tires you out, you know."

She looked at me quizzically, seeming ready to comment, but turned away quickly. I grabbed my water bottle and guzzled down another bellyful of liquid before following her to the locker rooms, praying disconcertedly that I would be able to survive another day of practice. Quarter mile days were the toughest, even when my blood sugar was normal – you had to maintain almost a 50m sprinting speed for the whole 400 metres. *God, how was I going to manage this?* Maybe I *should* invent some illness. Nah, I'll save that card for another day, today wasn't so bad. I'll just hang back with the rest of the slackers. Yeah, that sounds good.

Mom's car pulled up in front of the gymnasium 15 minutes after the grueling practice was over. I wrenched the backseat door open, threw my duffel bag on the floor of the minivan, and splayed myself across the seat. "Hi, Mom."

"Hi, kiddo." She glanced at me sideways while starting the engine. "Can you please sit up and strap up? I'm not moving until you do."

"All right, all right," I said, acquiescing. "Do you have any water in here?"

"Check in the back. You're looking a bit peaky – are you feverish?"

"No, its just the heat. Practice was pretty insane." I couldn't find any water behind the passenger seat.

"Well, make sure your sugars are under control, okay? The doctor said you wouldn't be able to run as well if they weren't within range."

"Can you get off my back already?! I told you they were fine." *Jeez.*

"I'm just saying. I never see you check yourself anymore, so I have no idea what's going on. You seem to be awfully lackadaisical about your diabetes stuff lately."

"Whatever, Mom. It's not like you watch me every second of the livelong day. I test my sugars, I give myself insulin, and I. Feel. Fine. I'm just tired from practice." I bent down to tie my sweaty shoelace, avoiding her eyes. "Stop badgering me."

"Where's your pump, then? I don't see it on your hip."

"Oh my GOD, what is this, a cross-examination?! I told you I can't run with it so I disconnect it during practice." *Damn, I left it under my pillow this morning. Hopefully she won't beat this to death…*

"Show it to me." *So much for that.*

"Uuum, no. Its tucked in between all my track sweats. I'll show it to you when we get home, unless you want me to rustle out all my smelly clothes." I pretended to open the zipper of my grimy duffel bag. "Be my guest." *I could pretend to stall, rifle around in here until we get home, when she'd be too distracted with dinner to care anymore.*

"No, fine. But I want to see you check your sugar in front of me when we get back."

"Have it your way. You're treating me like a common criminal, but what else is new?"

"You can victimize yourself all you want, but you'll do it, understood?"

"Right, of course. And after that, you can scour my room for weed, check my underwear drawer for condoms, and then give me a timeout in the kitchen corner for getting my multiplication tables wrong."

"Your defensiveness is very enlightening, I must say."

Just shut up. I threw her one last poisonous glance before glaring out the window until we pulled up in the driveway. I marched straight up to my room and slammed the door. She was in enough of a mood to check anything she knew or understood about my insulin junk. Which meant I had to take my pump, change the time back to 9:03am, and pretend to bolus myself 6 units for the toast and jam, milk and cornflakes I had eaten for breakfast before hustling to catch the chronically early bus. I repeated the same process for lunch and snack, attached it quickly to the infusion set on my stomach. I don't even know why I bother keeping an infusion set attached to myself – I never even use it. Suppose it was good for emergencies like this, though.

"Becky, get down here, and bring your kit!"

Down to the wire now. I couldn't possibly fabricate new times on my glucose monitor with the amount of time I had. I hurriedly splashed some calibration liquid on the strip and swaggered downstairs, feigning a casual attitude. "Here, you wanted to see my blood sugar? Totally normal, I told you. 122."

"Give me that." She snatched it from my hand and began to press a few buttons. I could feel the blood pounding in my ears – I knew she would try to check the glucose history. *Damn, damn, damn, she's not going to believe me. I'm absolutely done for this time. Crap, then Dad will come home and scream at me and threaten grounding or not letting me go to college and then I'll be completely done for...THINK!!! Come on...*

"Why are there no readings before this evening until three nights ago?"

I pretended not to hear, pouring myself a glass of Pepsi.

"REBECCA!"

"What?!"

"Where are all of your readings? There's only now, and then nothing dating back until Monday night. I KNEW you weren't checking!"

"MOM! Can you stop spazzing out? I never use this kit! I have one at school that I use since I'm there for a majority of the day." I paused, computing rapidly. "I usually keep it in my backpack but today we had to trade our uniforms in for laundry so I must have left it in my locker, which is why I had to use this one."

She frowned at me suspiciously, but I knew I had regained the upper hand. "What?! I can bring it home tomorrow if you want to be anal-retentive." I added a double eye roll for theatric effect and stormed out of the room. "WOW."

Victory.

Later that night I sat on my bed, my history materials strewn about me – study guides, notes, textbook, homework, laptop. I had gone over everything for the exam for the third time, but my brain was being porous again – randomly important facts would seem to wriggle through and escape until the next review sequestered them again. I sighed. I couldn't seem to concentrate either, I had to disconnect myself from the internet to avoid checking Gmail every 5 minutes or answering texts. But even then my mind would wander to the most mundane of details in meandering trains of thought, how I needed to put my lucky bracelet in my track bag for the sectional meet tomorrow, whether that dark stain on the wall was just a shadow from my lamp or actually black paint, and wondering what the term 'organic sea salt' actually meant. It didn't help that I had to extricate myself from the quagmire of exam materials every few hours to get a drink of water or use the bathroom. My stomach felt slightly pressured from all the water and food I had eaten.

I was completely worn out by the time 1am rolled around. *I can take a nap in study hall again,* I thought wearily as I trekked next door to brush my teeth and scour away the vestiges of Bavarian kreme donut that I had stashed away in my closet (along with Cheetos and a supply of Oreos that could probably satiate an entire Macedonian battalion). I looked at my reflection as the toothbrush traveled rhythmically under my cheeks. *Maybe Jen was right.* I'm really not entitled to look this haggard – gaunt, really. But the whole picture really brings out my eyebrows and cheekbones, doesn't it? I bent down over the sink to spit out the toothpaste, and out came a mouthful of blood. I ran my tongue tenderly over the raw spots on my gums, looking cursorily at my incisors in the mirror. The bleeding was getting worse, the borders of each tooth streaming rivulets of crimson liquid down onto my lip. I quickly gargled and sucked my cheeks together to tamponade the bleeding as I lumbered back to my room and flipped off the light. *Another day, another marathon completed.*

I caught snatches of sleep on Thursday night, waking intermittently and peering unthinkingly at the umbra of moonlight on my lampshade. A mild sense of panic was rising in my chest. The breathing was back.

The feeling wasn't like breathing during track practice, where you know the air will actually nourish your body if you obey the urge to breathe rapidly. Actually, it was as if I didn't need oxygen, but rather my body *didn't* need something else. Like it was using my breathing to get *rid* of something, to expunge some kind of poison, some noxium which had infiltrated my compromised system. I listened to my respirations as I faded in and out of consciousness, let my body take over the rise and fall of my chest: a rather sharp intake, and an alarmingly visceral exhale that seemed to derive straight from the depths of my lungs.

The breathing was enough to unsaddle my equanimity, but of course the problems didn't stop there. Would that the situation were so simple…No, whenever the breathing started, its malicious entourage inevitably followed. I don't know which of its minions frightened me the most: the palpitations that I couldn't calm and the sweating that would accompany them, the acid burning at the portal of my throat, the intermittent nausea that wasn't crippling enough to vomit but bad enough to induce acute wretchedness. And the thirst…like no thirst you could imagine – it was almost nonsensical, satirical, a caricature even of hyperglycemic thirst. Water itself begins to taste disgusting because your mouth resents the assault of ineffectual liquid, and you are relinquished, simply, to suffer through, swallowing through torturously desiccated tongue and lips.

I needed insulin soon, this I knew for a fact. But I was trapped.

Saturday was my cousin's graduation from law school, and we were all supposed to attend a huge celebration in his honor at this ritzy hotel in the city. Part of the festivities, of course, included a spectacular dinner buffet which I couldn't survive if I were expected to count calories, measure portion sizes, and persecute myself with thoughts of greater thigh circumference if I ate another salmon roll. Over and on top of that, the prom was next weekend, and there was no chance I was going to risk not fitting into my gown for an event I had waited 17 years to attend. I couldn't do any of it with insulin. I couldn't – I couldn't survive these next few days swelling up like a tomato and agonizing over my caloric intake and depriving myself of every element of gratuitous enjoyment that the last week of senior year embodied.

One more week, and then I'll put myself on insulin for good, I promised the ceiling, and God – if he were, in fact, somewhere above that whitewashed plaster. *Just one more, I promise. Just help me survive this last week, and after that I'll be healthy again, I'll give myself insulin no matter how bloated I feel, no matter how hungry, I'll never ever binge again. I'll get out of this rut, and I'll stop staring at the sky, I'll stop feigning control.* It'll be okay, it'll be okay, I whispered, I pleaded to myself as my alarm started to ring, this poisonous mantra which had never failed to fail. I don't know how many times I've prayed that prayer, entreated those entreaties, pledged those pledges, each successive set diluting the former in an iterative signature of destruction.

I walked to the bathroom for my general morning routine, feeling my heart start to pound – not out of nervousness but through some biologically derived rhythm hammering out its devilish cadence. *Right, gauntlet – here I come...*

I arrived at second period gym class with a splitting headache. We were in our volleyball unit, and every time I spiked the ball I felt like my brain was playing tennis against the vaults of my skull. Halfway through I absolutely couldn't endure the pulsating pain any longer, so I told my instructor that my head was hurting and could I please sit out for the remainder of the game. "Do you want to go to the nurse and ask for some Tylenol?" she asked, but I knew Tylenol would do squat. I politely declined and walked anemically over to the water fountain. I greedily sucked up enough water until my stomach hurt, then collapsed on the sidelines with my head gently resting in my hands.

"Hey hey," Nadia jogged up to kneel next to me for a few minutes, panting. "What's wrong?"

"Headache," I mumbled. "Stomachache. Sleep-deprived."

"Time of month, eh?" she said in a low voice.

I snorted. "No. Wish it were. That would make my life even more wonderful." I looked up at her and managed a weak grin. The truth was, I hadn't had a 'time of month' in over three years, but of course this was not exactly something to advertise. Judging from the cramps and mood swings and especially the bloating my friends were incessantly harping about, I honestly didn't feel as if I were missing much. Some days when I really considered the issue I would have liked the option to have children, but I was confident that when I got back on insulin the periods would come back.

We headed back to the locker room and changed back into street clothes. I always changed in the bathroom – I know everyone else had to strip down too, but somehow I felt that everyone was staring at me, at my legs, my stomach, my insulin pump scars, my flab and my bones. The stalls were infinitely less stressful. I walked out fully clothed over to my locker, but the 15 minutes of volleyball I had played had so drained me that I could barely muster the power to lift my backpack. My breathing was coming in shallow gasps as I walked feebly to my next class, pausing for a few seconds in the periphery of the hallway and leaning one hand against the lockers to catch a few deep breaths. *I need to eat something, give my body something to metabolize, that sometimes helps. I* have *to survive this week, I have to, have to.* When I arrived at the classroom, I unwrapped a granola bar and chewed it slowly, grateful for the saliva that momentarily rehydrated my mouth. After awhile, the urgent prompting to breathe calmed down and, relieved, I sat quietly until the bell rang.

Sixth period I was gasping again.

All right, I think I might need to bow out gracefully for some time, I obviously can't survive very long in this state. I began to negotiate frantically, my mind racing. Maybe if I give myself some insulin for the next few hours or days and drink a vat of water, I can flush out some of the ketones and offset this debilitating breathing. But the insulin would make me swell up again, and then how was I supposed to fit into my dress? Oh hellll... Well, maybe after I clear out some of the ketones then I can overeat until my blood sugar goes high, maybe that will offset the edema quickly. *Right, that sounds like a plan,* I mused as I leaned down towards my pump console and started punching in numbers.

The bus stopped at the corner of the road. I descended the stairs in a zombie-like trance, lifted my heavy head to look down the road to where my house lay in the distance. I imagined a rather melodramatic cinematic technique where the director targets one outstanding feature of the horizon's landscape and then pans out at 100mph in order to make the object appear ten times further away than it actually is. That was how my house seemed right now. In fact, my life at that moment was the panorama – and the camera was zooming out at a godforsaken speed, relinquishing me to the dust. I wanted to drop my backpack and splay out on the grass in defeat, admitting once and for all that this disorder was too insubordinate for me. But I took one step, sucked in a profound breath of air, another step, another gasp. Continuing these alternately until I arrived at the garage door, I punched in the code and staggered inside up to my bedroom. There, I collapsed on my bed, utterly spent.

Towards Healing

I don't know how long I slept. Oddly, I didn't wake up to pee or drink water. I wasn't even hungry, but my stomach's quiet rolling portended a serious ache. I could taste a nasty aroma in my mouth as I sat up, a sort of rotting sweetness, like alcoholic fumes from soured wine. My lips were so chapped that yawning cracked the skin at both ends and elicited stinging bleeds.

My mom was certainly making no secret of being behind schedule for dinner with her frenetic clanging down in the kitchen, haphazardly throwing together a quasi-edible dinner from one of those magazine recipe cards. Hastily, I splashed some water on my face and sluggishly went downstairs to the cacophonous kitchen, attempting to occlude my worsening stomachache by walking with my spine slightly hunched. *This long I've slept, and apparently all for nothing, I'm still as tired as I was.* I began to mechanically lay the plates and spoons out in their cursory arrangements. "Don't put one out for Ryan, he's going out bowling…Did you just wake up or something?" Mom said, catching a glimpse of my puffy face and my uncharacteristically indolent movements.

"Yeah, I didn't sleep last night at all, we had a huge calculus final today," I fibbed, too quickly. "Finish it off with a bang, they always say, right?"

She didn't hear me, having emitted a yelp of unprecedentedly high volume at dropping an open can of Roma tomatoes, which obligingly splattered on the cabinets and her professional pinstripe slacks. I took one look at the tomatoes and decided to skip dinner. If the meal involved anything relating to tomatoes, my acid reflux would soon be making an unsolicited appearance, and in this precarious state there was absolutely no way I was going to risk that. I probably wouldn't be able to hold down a meal anyway – my stomach was beginning to turn. "Need any help cleaning that up?" I asked her charitably, trying my best to perpetuate the act with a practiced poker face.

"No," she snapped. "Just try to stay out of my way."

"I'm actually just going to go upstairs and study. I'm really not that hungry anyway."

"Fine, go. I'm just going to nuke a Stouffer's for your father then."

The thick sense of nausea was beginning to envelop me – which I expected, but shakiness and dizziness and disorientation? *Seriously?* *HYPO*glycemia, on top of everything? I turned back to the staircase wearily, pulling each successive stair towards me by tugging the railings. I paused halfway up, head bowed, then ascended the remainder up to my bedroom. I quickly extracted my glucose monitor from the labyrinthine floor of clothes and books, and tested my sugar.

56!? Clearly I was too zealous with that insulin dose. The acid was accumulating in the back of my mouth, and I was having trouble differentiating it from the paralyzing waves of nausea that washed over me. I would be unable to eat anything sugary given the state of my stomach – I could barely swallow a few sips of apple juice without feeling like vomiting immediately. My brain was fading in and out of coherent thought – *will straw basketry make my blood sugar go up, should I start studying for history now, where did my turtles go* – WHAT? I don't even have turtles....

Grabbing the half-empty soda bottle on my dresser in a flash of determination, I attempted to quaff it in one go. I managed a few good sips but regretted them immediately, scrambling as rapidly as I could manage to the bathroom. There, I promptly threw up the soda as well as a few remnants of what seemed to be my lunch. The retching continued for about half a minute, opaque liquid dribbling viscously from the corners of my mouth. Starting to panic, I splashed water on my face and gently gargled with some tap water – there didn't seem to be any feasible way to get my sugar up without vomiting it all out again. *Maybe I should go to the ER. I should. I could go into a coma. I could faint right here on the bathroom floor.* But that would spell defeat, discovery, terminal disillusionment, and these were totally unacceptable.

I went to my bed and lay curled in a fetal position, shivering and almost delirious, trying desperately to think linearly out of the predicament. Contemplations were zigzagging through my head, undisciplined, willy-nilly, and the last I remembered was thinking that my mother's tulips shouldn't be in the middle of the lawn, and maybe I should water them with some orange juice, before oblivion mercifully overtook my jumbled brain. I dreamt no dreams, conjured no ephemera – my sleep was as black and uninspiring as the dead.

The entire night passed in that eviscerating pattern: I would wake up as my mouth filled with saliva – the immediate harbinger of upending vomit – grab the double-bagged garbage can next to my bed and regurgitate mostly speckled acid. After the heaving ceased, my mind would toe the line between sentience and unconsciousness, shutting down just as the nausea began to taper off. Gradually the interim between episodes lengthened – I was able to swallow more juice and the ache in my gut faded grudgingly away.

The next morning found me cocooned under my sheets, having overslept my alarm by more than half an hour. My muscles were limp and enervated, but my breathing was deep and nourishing, my stomach felt calm, and my brain was intelligible if slightly groggy. Mom barged into the room just as I was fading off to sleep again, her hair asunder with a comb in one talon and headband in the other.

"Becky you're *FTILL* in – what *if* that FMELL!!?" she shrieked, her voice muffled by the bobby pins protruding from her beak like a pincushion.

The garbage can I used to vomit was still perched next to my bed. *Damn, I should have disposed of that...*but it was entirely too late for damage control – she caught sight of it and whirled on me accusingly.

"What happened? Were you drinking?"

"'Course I was. Thursday night with finals next week, clearly I have nothing better to do." Somehow sarcasm didn't sound as trenchant when croaked through an arid tongue.

She felt my forehead, stroked my sweaty hair back from my forehead. I must have I looked like death, as her face lost all its thunderous fury in an instant.

"How do you feel? Why didn't you call me before?"

"Because of your interrogational penchant. Obviously, I was wrong."

She fell silent. I answered before she had a chance to begin her grilling again.

"It must have been something from the cafeteria yesterday. Barbecue beef. Always a tad sketchy." I glanced at her face surreptitiously. She wasn't buying it.

"I want you to test your blood sugar. Right now. In fact, you're not going to test it, I am." She looked around. "Where's your k-" She scooped up the monitor sitting on side table and grabbed one of my sallow hands from under the bedsheet, pricking a finger in painfully righteous determination.

"Its 272. I knew it was going to be high. "

High? 272?! HIGH?? I felt like laughing straight in her face. *Hah. Oh mother, mother dearest. If only you knew.* I did manage to omit a quiet snort.

She paused to consider. "Well, I suppose 272 isn't that bad, but the doctor says anything above 200 or 250 is going to make you feel rotten. You really should be testing more often if you want to avoid looking and feeling ill all the time. Which you do."

I grunted in irritation. "Okay, Mom, whatever. I told you it was something I ate."

"Well, obviously you can't go to school today. I'll call the dean's office and excuse you." She sighed and stood up, passing a hand wearily across her forehead. For a brief instant, I forgot my resentment, my irritation, weariness with my own travails to look at the whisper of pain crossing her face. What had I done to her, her peace of mind, her trust, her relationship with me and my dad and brother? To that smile now always tainted with smidgeons of cynicism and resigned concern, grief for a child that a mother could never feasibly express. It was now, for her, after all this ordeal and physical anguish, when I felt like crying.

"Stay in bed, you don't move." Her breath came out in a whoosh. "Well, I'm going to have to call work and tell them I can't come."

"You *really* don't have to. I'm okay now. Just tired."

"I'm going to bring you some chicken broth. You have your pump on?"

"Yeah, its on my stomach."

"You really need to start testing more frequently." I started to protest weakly again before she cut me off. "I don't want to hear it. Today I'm going to test you myself, I don't want any of your shenanigans. There's enough to worry about."

Easily fixed. She can do what she wants today. "Right, fine. Can you hand me my computer?"

She glanced at my laptop, glared at me in impregnated silence, then stalked out of the room. I sighed in relief, then nestled under the covers and fell into quiet sleep.

The remainder of the day I was an obedient diabetic. I ate vegetables and soup, I let Mom test my glucose levels, I gave myself insulin for every bite placed in my mouth. Rested, mostly, dreamt of little ketones swimming out into the toilet and blankets with patterns of Gatorade bottles. By evening I was restored enough to walk down the stairs to the kitchen to joke around with everyone for dinner. My pump was my staunch companion the entire day, faithfully injecting basals and boluses for the strict caloric intake I imposed for that period of normal blood sugars.

I retired early, feeling much stronger but still borderline debilitated. Everything had happened before, all the symptoms, the aches, the maladies, the trepidation, panic. And everything I had dealt with, convinced myself that I didn't need parents or emergency physicians or doctors or anyone. I was smart enough to create my illness, I was smart enough to perpetuate it without impediment, to cheat its consequences. Sure, there were times when I felt like throwing in the towel, but I was only human, yes? Everyone wants to admit defeat sometimes. But I was going to get better – I wanted to get better. Life isn't worth living without insulin. Sooner or later this is going to catch up with me. '*Because the house always wins. Play long enough, and the house takes you.*' I spoke to the ceiling again. *I'll do it. I can do it. It's been too long coming, from now on, it's the straight and narrow...*

The next morning I woke up with the sun glowing sardonically through my mesh window screens. Rubbing my eyes lazily, I went through my perfunctory morning routine and selected my combination of attire for the day. Unhooking my pump from the waistband of my pajamas while changing clothes was such an unfamiliar action – it was so often disconnected from my body that I barely remembered it existed. A new day had dawned, with fresh determination and raw grit. Checking my sugar (without any doctoring) before heading downstairs for breakfast was almost refreshing, and I faced the day with guns blazing and stallions charging, confident that I was larger than whatever diabulimia could throw at me.

I managed to last until lunchtime.

I'll do it tomorrow. Tomorrow, and I'll run with the baton – ad astra.

That was 4 years ago. Tomorrow still knocks on today's door, and yesterday – shackled and spent and disappointed – is still forced to answer.

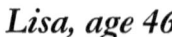

Lisa, age 46

The shrieking peal of my cell phone cut deftly through the humid silence of the car, leaving a frantic scrambling in its wake. Clutching the steering wheel tightly in my left hand, I fumbled around in my pocket until my fingers curled around the tiny vibrating nuisance and yanked it out. *Jane.*

"Hello?" I said, attempting my level best to be nonchalant.

"Hi, Mom."

"Where are you? You were supposed to be home over an hour ago, but I couldn't find you so I've gone off to Publix to get some groceries."

"Yeah, I'm sorry, something happened with the backstage crew, so rehearsal's gonna run late tonight. I'll catch a ride with Phil or something." There was a short pause. "Wait, did you say you were going to Publix?"

"There's no milk left, so I thought I'd finish off the shopping for the week."

"Can you get me a few litres of diet Coke and a packet of cheese pretzels? You know the ones where they dip them in that chipotle coating."

"I don't know, hun, can't you eat something…better? Like yogurt? Or vegetables? Cheese pretzels are hardly diabetes fare."

I swear you can *hear* teenagers roll their eyes over the phone. "Throw some apples in there, then."

"The next time you plan on being late at rehearsal, make sure you tell me. I know you laugh at how much I freak out, but try being considerate."

"Bye, Mom. Thanks for the pretzels."

I sighed and tossed the phone into the coffee holder. It wasn't so much 'freaking out' as it was a constant whisper of worry, an insidious undertone of calamity that always managed to worm itself between the sheaves of my waking hours. I desperately wished there was something I could do myself, rip out my own pancreas and live with the shots and the counting and the weight gain and the testing and all the daily perturbances that she had to endure. But she was a 'special' diabetic in addition to those injustices. Hah. 'Special' diabetic. Even that phrase sounded redundant in my head, kind of like saying 'an orange orange' or a 'dry desert'...

Jane was always on the slightly plump side – never fat, but never skinny either. The closest she came to slim was the few weeks before she was diagnosed. But then, slim is too politically correct a description. She was gaunt, haggard without emaciation, with sunken eyes and anemic cheeks. I thought at first that she was trying some radical new diet, which wouldn't have been implausible considering her penchant for weight loss gimmickry. Whatever it was, I thought, it was working – she shed a startling amount of weight in quite a short time. I even remember complimenting her during the first few weeks – before her clothes started hanging from her body, before she became sluggish and disenchanted and obsessed with her body and her clothes and her dress size. I told her she looked beautiful and stylish, and what was she doing and maybe I should try it too.

But if I could go back in time and modify anything in my life, I would take back those words. Because I realize now what she thought I was saying, what I should have realized what was implicit in those carelessly selfish and materialistic words. That she wasn't beautiful before she lost all of that weight, and how she thought I didn't value her until she was streamlined enough to fit into fashionable clothes, that body shape was the ultimate culmination of restraint and discipline. Oh, I know that there were many other things that factored into it, but somehow I feel she thinks I betrayed her. And it's difficult for me, sometimes, to believe that I did not.

After she was diagnosed, all the weight came back within a few days. She even put on a few extra pounds. But I didn't even think about how her body changed, because there was such an overwhelming amount of information to absorb post-diagnosis, with endocrinologists and dieticians and nurses knocking incessantly on our door to hand out helpful sheets of information that we would eventually be able to recite backwards. I should have known, figured out that her depressed moods after leaving the hospital weren't just due to the enormous burden of the new diagnosis, but also to those 20 pounds which had been so abruptly plastered on her recently trim frame. Even our endocrinologist at the time recommended that we see a psychologist, as she seemed so 'down and out.'

I wish it had ended there, but things are never that simple. Our entire family was so focused on insulin injections and lancets and alcohol swabbing – the damned minutiae, and then the divorce – that nobody bothered to parse out what was going on inside her head rather than her bloodstream. The thorn of weight gain seemed to be so deeply embedded that little else regained its proper context after her diagnosis. I can't imagine the mental oppression she must have undergone while her father and I were managing her diabetes care, and I wish I could say that she eventually regained her largely cheerful demeanor. But I can't, and unless you've experienced it for yourself, you cannot know how that change can torture a mother.

I think she actually started to vomit first, before doing anything with her insulin. (I can't know for sure, because she vacillates between freely admitting these things to me, and denying them completely. But based on what she's said during moments of spontaneous divulging, I believe this might be true.) I noticed some odd aberrations in her blood sugars even when I was still monitoring her myself, but never gave much thought to the cause. Her HbA1c levels were reasonable during that time, but once we let her go on the pump, the values rose spectacularly.

Anyway, the details aren't terribly important. All I know is that before she was diagnosed, she lost a drastic amount of weight, and now she sometimes doesn't take insulin for the same reason. I would force her to go see a psychiatrist or a therapist, but she's actually a high-functioning high-schooler. I'm sure they'd take one look at her stats and send us packing.

I turned the corner into our subdivision, where I caught a glimpse of the tail end of the blue garbage truck disappearing around the other end of the street. *Damn, she must have forgotten to put out our trash,* I thought, hitting the accelerator. Jerking abruptly into our driveway, I sprinted inside and collected the plastic bags of trash from the first floor receptacles and dumped them into the master garbage bin to be laid out on the sidewalk for the truck's convenience. As I carried it outside, a flash of unfamiliar bright vermillion caught my eye, and I gingerly poked around inside the bag until I found the source. *McDonald's?* Nobody from our family eats from the golden arches, really, unless…my shoulders slumped. Not again. Please.

Maybe she wasn't omitting again. Maybe Brian just decided to grab a quick dinner with his friends. But he hates McDonald's – says they taste like pulverized plastic and expired potatoes. I gently shook the bag around to attempt looking inside the incriminating container. *Damn, damn, damn.* Fritos packages, Twinkie wrappers, inundating amounts of pudding cups, even some balled-up ice cream foils. And that was only one small sample – who knew what other travesties were lurking at the bottom of the vessel.

How was this possible!? She seemed to be doing so well, I saw her testing her blood sugar and changing her pump sets. Maybe these were old, maybe she was just clearing out her closet of old sins from months or weeks ago. God, I hope it wasn't just weeks. No, it can't be, I'm just psyching myself out. I'll ask her when she gets home. Or perhaps I won't ask her, I'll just watch a little closer than before, maybe she'll tell me herself. *But she won't, you know it.*

Dejected, I paced around in the kitchen, absentmindedly rubbing scuff marks from the linoleum floor. For lack of anything better to do, I reheated some chicken pasta from the previous night and booted up my computer, burying myself in numbers and spreadsheets to abstain from agonizing over the Jane dilemma, simply waiting for her to return home.

I heard keys in the back door at about 11pm, when she noisily scraped the mud from her galoshes and tossed her slicked jacket on one of the kitchen chairs. I listened as best as I could from the den office – what was she removing from the fridge and rustling around in the cupboards? Did she test her sugar before starting to munch? I couldn't expressly hear any evidence of diabetes – no staccato click of the lancet punching through skin, no beeping of the kit or pump. I suppose it doesn't have to mean much, today could be one of those singular days where these overworked high-schoolers just come home and eat everything in sight.

"Jane?"

I heard her move quickly in alarm. "Mom? What are you still doing awake?"

"Couldn't sleep, those baristas must have given me a caffeinated blend this evening instead of my regular decaf."

"How was your day?" she asked, strolling into the room. Her hands were notably empty.

"Same old, deadlines creeping up. I noticed you didn't take the garbage out today." I watched her reaction in my peripheral vision, where her small jerk of unease was quickly obtunded by her pretense of turning away to examine the statuette of a shepherd on the bookcase. "Anyway, I did it, so just remember next time."

No response. Honestly, I didn't know what to make of her silence, but things weren't looking encouraging. She was too quiet for any potential lack of compunction.

"Sorry, I totally forgot."

"Rehearsal go okay? Did you have dinner?"

"Well, Sam baked a tray of brownies, so I ate one of those, but I'm still kinda hungry."

"There's some leftover pasta in the fridge." I heaved myself out of the armchair with a few joints creaking along the way. "I'm going to bed. Night, hun."

She walked over to kiss me on the cheek. "G'night, Mom." Her breath wafted a sickeningly sweet-sour smell as she turned to walk into the kitchen. *Has she been drinking? What IS that? And what, you ate a* brownie*?!*

She told me once, in a moment of self-preservation, that I should be wary of times when I found her eating like a normal person. I should be suspicious if she didn't nitpick over calories or fuss over portions or time her mealtimes obsessively. I should start to wonder if she didn't exercise religiously in the mornings, if she showed no qualms about going out at odd times of the day. If she seemed reckless, in general, buying things that she normally wouldn't, saying things that she would never utter. Uninhibited, was what she said. "I know it sounds weird, unbelievable even, but if I start acting like a normal teenager then you know something's up..." Straight from the horse's mouth, and yet I still rebelled. Because part of being a parent entails *wanting* your kid to be normal, to fit in and be part of the symphony of their generation. Idealism is rubbish. Nobody wants their child to follow the proverbial unique drumbeat, unless they themselves can set the cadence. And sometimes we want this normality, or fettered individuality, so much that we actually end up believing that it is reality.

I closed my eyes and drifted off, under the hum of the quiet corner radiator. I saw the bathroom light flip on before I finally fell asleep.

"Mom? Mom! Wake up!" Blissful Saturday mornings were always tainted by Jake's inopportune screeching, usually intended to inform me that he had to be chauffeured to his father's house for their weekend bonding session. Baseball. *Ugh.*

I groaned. "God, can't you drive yourself," and pulled the covers over my ears.

"OOO can I can I?? Sweet! JANE!! Guess what?"

"Oh be quiet." I peered at the clock through the vise I had created with the comforter, then grudgingly abandoned the covers and put my slippers on. "Did you have your cereal?"

"Uh...no, you promised to make pancakes and bacon this morning, remember?"

"You could have finished by now, just stick a few Pop-tarts in the toaster and have a glass of OJ. We're already running late."

"But there aren't any left, and the orange juice is over too. You won't let me microwave the bacon because it's TOO messy." He glared at me sternly, his voice adopting a certain whiny quality. "The only thing you'll let me do is toast a Pop-tart and butter a slice of bread, and the marmalade is over too. I'm really starving."

"How is it possible that there aren't any Pop-tarts left? I bought an army-sized crate just last week – that was supposed to last for the next month!"

"Jane eats all of them." He paused to consider his incriminating strategy. "Sometimes she has them for dinner. Aren't Pop-tarts only for breakfast?"

"All right, I can't deal with this right now. Go downstairs and make yourself a PB&J while I get ready." I grabbed a pair of pants and a T-shirt hastily, shaking my head and muttering in disbelief. "A week-and-a-half! An entire Costco box! Jeez, I swear you kids have to cut down your junk food intake. One box!"

I stumbled into the hallway, attempting to pull on a pair of mismatched socks. Of course I didn't believe that Jake had no part in it, but something nagged disconcertingly at the back of my brain…My eyes on the dusty floor, I collided with something in the aperture to Jane's room.

"JANE, WAKE – oh, you're already awake. Get ready, I need to drop Jake at Dad's. Are you going?"

Her eyes darkened slightly. "No, I'm good, thanks. Can you drop me at the train station on the way, though?"

"Where are you going?"

"We're meeting downtown. Hanging out. We might catch the free jazz concert in the evening."

"That's nice. You should visit your dad sometimes, though, hun. Did you pack some lunch or dinner?"

"Nah, I'll just buy a Potbelly's or something – we'll probably end up eating at a restaurant."

Huh.

"Take your kit, yeah?"

"Mmhmm." She turned back to her dresser. "Are you still making pancakes for breakfast?"

"No, you guys can grab something from the pantry. Oh, and speaking of the devil, how IS it that all the Pop-tarts are *over*?! How many of them do you galosh every day?"

"How many do I ea – you think *I* finished them?"

"You're brother certainly vehemently denies it."

"Right, and he's the paradigm of sainthood. Have you SEEN him lately? He's always eating something."

"Great! So it wasn't him, and it wasn't you. Unless I'm eating in my sleep, we must have a terrible gnome problem."

"Awww, Mom, don't let's be silly. Gnomes only eat corn dogs. It's those pesky leprechauns – they go totally haywire over Pop-tarts."

I scowled, trying to claw at my irritation but feeling it begin to dissipate. "Wait till you start grocery shopping for yourself, then you'll understand how frustrating it is when your wayward children eat all the junk food while the bell peppers and broccoli are growing fungus."

"MOOOOOOMMM? There's a huge package by the door! Should I bring it in?" Jake yelled from the foyer.

"Yes please – who's it from?"

"Lil…lillu…LILLY?"

"OH! Jane, your insulin must be here."

"Cool."

"Unpack it and put it in the fridge when you go downstairs. And hurry up, Jake and I are leaving in five minutes."

"Coming, coming!" She ran to the bathroom and slammed the door shut.

243

I trudged up the steps to the front door after returning from the train station, pausing to rearrange the motley pots on the windowsill. The first thing I saw when I opened the front door was the Lilly package lying smack dab in the center of the foyer tiles. Ugh. *Jane, I thought I told you to put those inSIDE!* Annoyed, I retrieved the razor blade from the office desk drawer and extracted the tiny vials of insulin from beneath the ice packs and Styrofoam peanuts, wedging the refrigerator door open with my ankle. I opened the rotating door of the butter compartment allotted for medications, expecting a neat cavity where I could stack the new bottles. Instead, it was overflowing left, right, and center – not with Tylenol, probiotics, or Jake's inhaler – but innumerable bottles of crimson-labeled insulin. *What is going on?* The prescription said 2 bottles per month, right? Why are there so many left behind?...*I haven't checked this drawer in so long, maybe some of them are empty.* I rustled around. Only one was uncapped, and I snatched it for examination. *What? Expiration date was over 2 months ago?!*

I shook my head, perplexed. Of course, she might have required less insulin for that low-carb temporary diet craze of hers. Or she might need smaller doses – Dr. Bruni said that losing weight could shrink insulin requirements, and Jane did seem to have lost a few pounds recently. *I don't know what I'm thinking. I don't even know what I want to think. Does she seriously need to beat me over the head – why am I being so damn recalcitrant?*

What do you do when trust isn't even the issue? What do you do when the infinitesimal gap between trust and gullibility is so thoroughly manipulated that you can't see past your own nose, the forest for the trees, the analogy for the idiom? What if she isn't taking insulin again, and I've been too thickheaded and too blindsided by my fear of what might be true to actually grasp the peril?

And if she is doing what I think she is, what do I do then? Confront her, scream at her, throw things? Go on the warpath? I know those aren't going to work. I've tried. I've forced her to go to the doctor – they just told her to see a psychiatrist for depression, and upped her insulin doses to fix the HbA1c. I've given her shots myself, obsessively watched her glucose monitor, but I can't do that all the time, can I? I've told her that she'll go on dialysis, that she won't be able to get married and have kids, that she'll be so incapacitated that she'd *wish* for the opportunity to take care of herself. Because it passes, that window of clemency, and soon even human efforts do little to dampen the inexorable processes that our bodies foist upon ourselves. Hell, I've even told her that she's going to die, and she just looked back at me with… I don't know what she felt – maybe defiance, nonchalance, scorn, charitable attention. But I saw some humanity in there, I know it. I saw a microscopic flash of fear, sorrow, guilt, *anguish* most of all – in that spark she thought I couldn't perceive. Cue the cellos, the heartrending soprano violin and the melancholy bass, the ones I could hear on her behalf. At times I just want to grab her by the shoulders and shake the living daylights out of her, compel her to hear those strains of tragedy. But would it make any difference, I wonder…

Both of them returned early in the evening – Jake's dad dropped him off, and told me to say hello to Jane, he was sorry he had missed her. Jake started to open one of the cabinets with his grimy post-soccer paws, but I fielded him towards the bathroom to have a shower amidst acute protest. "No 'aawwwwws' or buts about it. Now. Otherwise no pizza for dinner."

"PIZZA?!"

"Yeah, I'm sorry for not making pancakes this morning. You guys get a treat tonight."

"Yeeeaaahh!! Thanks, Mom, you're the best!" He scrambled away upstairs, and I sat on the kitchen table to quietly read the Saturday paper.

Jane lumbered downstairs and sat down in the chair beside me with a bottle of cerulean-hued nail polish. "How was your day?"

I set aside the newspaper, watching the rod pace the length of her nail in precise strokes. "Regular. Nothing fascinating, did some cleaning and cooking. How was yours?"

"It was fun, I guess. We ended up waiting, like, *two hours* at the train station for David. But we got to go to this free flamenco demonstration at the Cultural Center, which was really cool. And they were giving away free plastic castanets!"

"Was there a flamenco guitarist?" I paused, looking at the nail polish for the first time. "My God, that's a really ghastly color." She smirked and rolled her eyes, lifting her hand up to examine the precision of her painting. It was then that I noticed something odd.

"Not sure about bona fide, but he seemed pretty good. Really fast." There were no flecks of brown on the tips of her fingers anymore. None. Completely blanched and white, smooth, just like mine.

I recall the day when she came to me, thumb bleeding because she had tried to excise the calloused and pocked skin with a clumsy nail clipper. *The lancet isn't going through anymore – FOUR TIMES, four times and still no blood,* she had hissed angrily, and I can't forget the poisonous gaze of her eyes. *What did I do? Why is she looking at me like that?* I remember thinking. I had taken her hand and bandaged it, running my unsullied finger sadly across hers and seeing the tiny speckled scars clustered in the thickened skin around her nails.

"Hmmm? Bona fide, huh. Hmm. Jane, can you –?" I stopped abruptly. *What? Can you – tell me? Can you – come clean? Can you – help me understand?* What was I supposed to say to not make her clam up? How do we get out of this long catch-22?

My thoughts were interrupted by a staccato series of beeps, which ceased as suddenly as they started. I heard Jane mutter under gritted teeth, as she angled her head towards her right side to glance at her hip.

"S'wrong?"

"Uhhh...my pump is low on insulin." She turned her attention back towards her nails, glancing up at me quickly. "It likes to chirp about that."

"Well, go and refill it, then. I swear to God I've heard that beep for at least a week. Maybe more."

"I don't really need to do it now, there's a few units left."

246

"Jane…"

"What? Let me deal with it, okay?"

"Well, we're having pizza for dinner, so make sure you have enough insulin in there to cover it. You probably have to give a square wave for pizza, right? All that cheese?"

"I guess. Whatever. There should be enough left for a few slices."

I sighed and got up from the table.

Jake noisily slurped up the vestiges of his lemonade, and reclined back in his chair dramatically. "Now THAT's what you call dinner." He rubbed his belly cartoonishly. "I vote we have it every night."

"Fat chance, kiddo. Clean up your place, please."

"Jake, it's your turn to do the dishes," Jane said, between bites.

"Uh, no, what?! I did them yesterday!"

"No, that was me, definitely. I remember scrubbing your greasy plate with all the crusted macaroni." She glared at him. "Took me 10 minutes. For one stupid plate."

"Uh, first of all, we didn't even *have* dinner here last night, and second – WHAT macaroni? We never had macaroni, are you crazy?"

I shot her an odd look between clearing the napkins. "Jake's right – what macaroni? We never ate macaroni."

"Moooom, she's just trying to get out of doing the dishes!"

Jane looked confused. "Oh…I thought we had mac'n'cheese yesterday… but where'd we eat then?"

"UM, Grandma's?! What is WRONG with you?"

"Oh…riiiight. But didn't we have macaroni there?"

"No. Nimrod. She baked a Bolognese just for you, remember?"

She frowned, and I watched as realization slowly dawned on her face. She chuckled sheepishly. "Yeah, sorry. Don't know why I forgot about that."

"You're forgetting a bunch of stuff lately. Like the garbage." I turned back to the sink. "And you were supposed to have mopped the floor last night, it's still dirty."

Jane pushed back her chair abruptly. "Yeah, sorry. All these European history factoids are crowding out the important stuff." She yawned loudly and pushed in the chair, bumping into the edge of the table rather haphazardly. "Man, I'm stuffed. Gonna go take a quick nap on the couch. Wake me up in 30? I'll do the dishes then, after they soak properly."

"I'll wake you up *now*," Jake growled, as she trudged off to the living room.

An hour later, I remembered with a start that Jane was still asleep. *Damn, she's going to kill me. She should have woken herself up – she gets entirely too much sleep anyway. Always napping. Teenagers.*

I walked to the couch in the adjacent room and reached out with my arm to jolt her awake, but stopped just as my fingers touched her shoulder. I stood still for a few seconds, listening to her sonorous breathing. It was quiet, unobtrusive – melodious even. Hearing the sound might be calming for anyone who couldn't see her at the same time, watch in growing panic as her chest rose and fell with a profundity that I had never seen before. She wasn't gasping, but they were too deep and too long, as if she were straining the very edges of her lungs with each intake. I leaned in with a start.

"JANE! Wake up!" My voice, even to me, sounded frantic, as I grasped her shoulder and rattled it around.

"Mgrnadnh," was her incoherent reply.

"Are you still congested from last week? Your breathing sounds really, *really* weird."

"Mmmyah lil' bit Mom I told you to wake me up in half an hour," she mumbled, turning on her back to face the other side of the La-Z-boy.

"Jane! It's been more than an hour. Be grateful I let you sleep this long – you need to do the dishes and also mop the floor since you didn't do it yesterday."

"Okayokayokay. Man, time flies."

"…When you're sleeping. Right, we know. Get on with it."

I came back to the kitchen twenty minutes later to find her leaning on the mop, gulping down a glass of water. I surveyed the floor in mild irritation.

"This is all you've done?"

She glanced up at me in mild surprise. "What? I finished."

"You wha – finished?? Oh, no you don't," I snapped, as she made to toss the bucket of mop water in the sink. "Look there. And here. And here by the cabinet. There's still so many stains." I glared at her. "Back to work. Now."

"It's so unfair that I have to do the entire floor by myself. And these stains are so tough," she whined, scouring at a particularly conspicuous one in front of the sink. After a few seconds of rather anemic scrubbing, she bowed her head and paused to catch her breath.

I sighed. "It's mopping, Jane, not marathon running. Just finish it, yeah? Without dramatics, I want to see all of those marks gone by the time I get back."

"'Kay I'm done." She stomped into the living room half an hour later. "You can do your military inspection now."

249

"Jane, can you come and sit down for a second?"

She raised an eyebrow and complied, looking at me with a typical teenage wariness. "What's up?"

"Are you okay?"

A shadow flitted across her face, and I could see the beginnings of that intentionally blank look she would adopt to allay any misgivings.

"I'm...fine, why?"

"I don't know. You're just...not yourself. You don't laugh anymore. You're always tired and pale and I feel like I'm losing you to something."

"Mom. Please. I'm fine. It's your job to worry, you wouldn't be normal if you didn't."

"Are you sure you're taking care of yourself?" *The direct approach.* She knew exactly what I was referring to.

"Yah." Not quite a statement, not quite an exclamation.

We sat in silence for a few seconds, me watching the pillow on the other side of the couch, and she watching me equally as quietly.

"Mom?"

I looked up at her wearily. I'm sure my eyes were pleading, but I couldn't bring myself to care. "Yeah."

"Can I go? I have to study for my history midterm."

I shrugged. "It's up to you." Every fiber screamed at me to grill her, to pin her down and extract a confession so I could fix her, make her well. But I couldn't. I didn't want to lose Jane in addition to Jane's body.

I watched her as she turned the corner to the staircase walk down the dimly lit hallway to the staircase. *Sometimes though, I felt as if I were losing both...*

RESOURCES

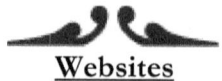
Websites

Diabulimia Helpline
www.diabulimiahelpline.org
(1ˢᵗ and only non-profit organization in the United States dedicated to diabulimia support)

Diabetics With Eating Disorders (DWED)
http://www.dwed.org.uk/
(Non-profit organization in the United Kingdom for ED-DMT1 support)

Diabulimiahelpline and DWED are sister sites. Both have Facebook support groups/forums – contact the support pages on the websites for more information.

GraceNutrition
http://www.gracenutrition.org/index.php
(Grace Shih, RD, MS is a private practice dietician in California, author of the first book about diabulimia, with extensive experience in treatment of patients with diabetes and eating disorders)

Ramey Nutrition
http://www.rameynutrition.com/
(Scarlett Ramey and her nutrition clinic take unique and effective approaches towards patient care in that they address overarching aspects of an individual's treatment regimen; they are experienced in treating diabetes and eating disorders)

Defeat Diabulimia
http://www.diabulimia.info
(Author's website, basic information about diabulimia, support, links, and contact information)

Blogs

(A few of the following have not been updated for an extended period, but it is at times helpful to read the chronological narratives of former patients)

The Butter Compartment
http://www.thebuttercompartment.com/

Diabulimia SOS
http://diabulimiasos.weebly.com/support.html

Diabolical Diabulimia
http://crosshatched.wordpress.com/about/

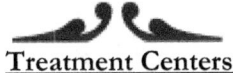

Treatment Centers

(These centers have rehabilitation programs designed specifically for diabulimia patients, unlike many other inpatient/outpatient therapies)

Center of Hope for the Sierras in Reno, NV
http://centerforhopeofthesierras.crchealth.com/

Casa Palmera Institute in Del Mar, CA
http://casapalmera.com/diabulimia-symptoms-and-treatment/

Cumberland Hospital for Children and Adolescents in New Kent, VA
http://cumberlandhospital.com/chronic-illness/diabetes-and-eating-disorders/

Park Nicolette Melrose Institute in Minneapolis, MN
http://www.parknicollet.com/medical-services/eating-disorders

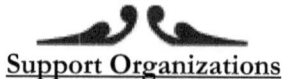

Support Organizations

Juvenile Diabetes Research Foundation (JDRF)
www.jdrf.org

American Diabetes Association (ADA)
www.ada.org

National Eating Disorders Association (NEDA)
http://www.nationaleatingdisorders.org/

Books

*DIABULIMIA: Diabetes + Eating Disorders; What It Is and How to Treat It:
A Guide for Individuals and Families*
By Grace Shih, RD, MS
CreateSpace Independent Publishing Platform

Eating to Lose: Healing from a Life of Diabulimia
By Maryjeanne Hunt
Demos Health Pub

AUTHOR'S NOTE

Dear Reader:

Thank you sincerely for taking the time to peruse through this book. My hope is that – despite your particular background and reasons for reading it – you have garnered snippets of knowledge about diabulimia which might aid in its overall cognizance. Although progress has been accomplished in leaps and bounds, it is still a grossly misunderstood and misrecognized condition. The tragedy is that if diabulimia is recognized early, many of its complications can be prevented – it is this goal towards which we strive today. There are many amazing individuals – patients, physicians, nurses, dieticians – working tirelessly for its eradication. It is my ultimate wish that this piece of writing contributes an iota to that body of work, a different perspective on the illness from a former patient with medical training.

As you might have surmised, the reflections preceding each chapter are my own. I was diagnosed with Type I diabetes at the age of 11, and struggled with diabulimia for almost 10 years. Like many other patients, I underwent incessant cycles of relapse and remission, each successive one worse than its precedent. Unfortunately, it was a long time before I received proper treatment and counseling (during my undergraduate years) – I didn't think it was necessary given that I was relatively functional. As such, I later went on to receive an undergraduate degree in chemistry, and then entered medical school. I believed my journey with the illness might provide a unique insight into some of the social aspects of diabulimia that might not be immediately accessible to healthcare practitioners. It was my hope to contextualize and synthesize such knowledge with the pathophysiological, evidence-based, and clinical principles gleaned during medical training.

Do not do what I did, do not stall in terms of treatment – there are too many wasted years, too many forfeited relationships, too many complex cognitive frustrations. It is difficult, and at times the least you can do is to grit your teeth, look up, and keep walking. But believe this: recovery is possible – and if you relentlessly believe in yourself, your patient, your friend, sibling, daughter or son – then there is no question that you (or they) can ultimately defeat this illness.

Aarti E. Sharma
Stanford Medical School
MD candidate, Year 4

Author biography:

Aarti Sharma holds a bachelors of science in chemistry from the University of Illinois, Chicago. She is a former recipient of the Barry M. Goldwater Scholarship, American Scandinavian Foundation Grant, and Endocrine Society NIH Research Grant. She is currently a fourth-year medical student at the Stanford University School of Medicine, where she is a recipient of the MedScholars research award and the co-editor-in-chief of H&P: The Stanford Medical School Journal.

ACKNOWLEDGEMENTS

Special acknowledgement to the Stanford MedScholars program for their generous monetary support.

Dr. Ann Goebel-Fabbri, who works tirelessly for the subject of diabetes and eating disorders in multiple venues – she is known to many diabulimia patients and her help through editing and interview is a true testament to her dedication.

Dr. Laura Bachrach, who was the catalyst for this project, encouraging the concept throughout the initial stages despite my own misgivings. Her advice, support, and genuine care throughout medical school have been invaluable.

Dr. Kathy Eckert, whose lecture at Stanford was another stepping stone, and who helped me understand so many nuances of diabulimia – not the least of which was the necessity to propagate its clinical recognition.

Dr. Audrey Shafer, who has been a source of literary education since my first year of medical school, advising me regarding the publishing process, and editing the included epigrams. Without her advocacy through the Stanford Biomedical Ethics and Humanities program, this project would not have been possible.

Dr. Larry Zaroff, a wonderful humanities professor who instilled the importance of the patient perspective, and who helped with editing the field narratives.

Dr. Tina Cowan, one of my clinical biochemistry professors, who clarified molecular complexities of the diabulimia state and generously helped with the pathophysiology section.

Scarlett Ramey, a dietician truly dedicated to not only the nutritional but also psychological equanimity of her patients. She is one of the few clinicians who understands what traverses through the mind of a diabulimia patient, and has been nothing but supportive.

Dr. Nounou Taleghani, my Educator-4-Care and mentor at Stanford, who is a consistent source of humor and provided insightful suggestions for the book format.

Dr. James Lock, who generously helped to connect me with knowledgeable faculty, as well as provided feedback on relevant psychiatry material.

Dr. Stesha Doku, one year my senior in medical school – an amazing graphic designer who did all the work and photography for the covers.

Maryjeanne Hunt, who wrote the first narrative book on diabulimia and previewed the book – a writer truly committed to solidarity and a concrete testament to palpable recovery.

And last but certainly not least, **Dr. Marina Basina** – my dedicated mentor through the course of this entire project. She is the paradigm of diabetologists – tirelessly committed to both her clinical duties as well as research and charitable work. I have learned so much from her these past 4 years, and hope one day to become as excellent, generous, and compassionate a clinician as she is.

Heartfelt thanks to all the other countless clinicians who lent their expertise and clinical insights. Whether it be a word, a sentence, or a chapter derived from your narratives, I appreciate the time you dedicated despite your busy clinical/research obligations. I truly hope that your experiences were translated effectively into this volume.

To all of the patients and families who I cannot name here: know this – we will triumph. Thank you all for contributing towards that endeavor, each and every one of you in your own way.